Student Study Resource:
Study Outlines, Solutions to
Odd-Numbered Problems and Ready Notes

for use with

Accounting:
What the Numbers Mean

Fifth Edition

David H. Marshall
Millikin University - Emeritus

Wayne W. McManus
International College of the Cayman Islands

Daniel F. Viele
Webster University

Ready Notes Prepared by
Martha Pointer
East Tennessee State University

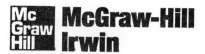 **McGraw-Hill**
Irwin

Boston   Burr Ridge, IL   Dubuque, IA   Madison, WI   New York   San Francisco   St. Louis
Bangkok   Bogotá   Caracas   Kuala Lumpur   Lisbon   London   Madrid   Mexico City
Milan   Montreal   New Delhi   Santiago   Seoul   Singapore   Sydney   Taipei   Toronto

McGraw-Hill Higher Education

A Division of The McGraw-Hill Companies

Student Study Resource: Study Outlines, Solutions to Odd-Numbered Problems and Ready Notes
for use with
ACCOUNTING: WHAT THE NUMBERS MEAN
David H. Marshall, Wayne W. McManus and Daniel F. Viele

Published by McGraw-Hill/Irwin, an imprint of the McGraw-Hill Companies, Inc., 1221 Avenue of the Americas, New York, NY 10020. Copyright © 2002 (1999, 1996, 1993, 1990) by the McGraw-Hill Companies, Inc. All rights reserved.

1 2 3 4 5 6 7 8 9 0 QPD/QPD 0 9 8 7 6 5 4 3 2 1

ISBN 0-07-247598-6

www.mhhe.com

NOTE TO STUDENT:

Your textbook is the principal resource that will contribute to your success in the course for which it was purchased. Other resources include your instructor, your classmates, your study efforts, and the supplements that accompany the text. These supplements are:

- **Student Study Resource: Study Outlines, Solutions to Odd-Numbered Problems, and Ready Notes.** This volume is designed to accelerate your learning and to improve your performance in the course. The *Study Outlines* emphasize the key ideas, key points, key relationships, and key terminology that we believe are critical to your learning and retention. The *Study Outlines* eliminate the need to copy information from transparencies or PowerPoint presentations, and provide space for you to take class notes. You may find it worthwhile to review the information contained in these outlines even if your instructor does not use them in class on a regular basis. The *Solutions to Odd-Numbered Problems* provide full solutions (not just check figures) for all odd-numbered exercises and problems in the text. Even-numbered problems are usually similar to the preceding odd-numbered problem. Having the full solution to the preceding exercise or problem available as a model provides additional examples beyond those in the text, reinforces learning, minimizes frustration, and facilitates your study efforts. The *Ready Notes* are reduced-sized copies of the Ready Shows (PowerPoint® slides) that some instructors may use when making classroom presentations; as with the *Study Outlines*, space is provided for your note taking.

- **Study Guide and Working Papers.** The *Study Guide* contains chapter outlines, review questions (matching, true-false, and multiple choice) with explanatory answers, and short exercises with solutions. *Working Papers* are set up for each problem in the text to facilitate your approach to the correct solution and to eliminate "busy work." Student reviews of this supplement from the first four editions of the text have been highly favorable and quite encouraging. You can order a copy of the *Study Guide and Working Papers* volume through your bookstore, or by calling McGraw-Hill at **1-800-338-3987**. When placing your order, ask for **ISBN** 0-07-247523-4.

The appendix of the text is a copy of Intel Corporation's 1999 Annual Report. For investor information, including annual reports, 10-K and 10-Q reports, or other financial literature (all of which is provided without cost), contact Intel's agent and registrar:

Harris Trust & Savings Bank
311 West Monroe, P.O. Box A3504, Chicago IL 60690-3504 USA
Call **1-800-298-0146** (U.S. or Canada) or **(312) 360-5123** (worldwide) for annual report ordering.

You are encouraged to visit Intel's World Wide Web site at: *http://www.intel.com.* Specific information of interest to investors can be found at: *http://www.intc.com.* The website for this textbook, *http://www.mhhe.com/business/accounting/marshall5e* also provides links to Intel and other real-world examples used in the problem materials.

Contents

ACCOUNTING IS THE PROCESS OF:

· IDENTIFYING, · MEASURING, and · COMMUNICATING	ECONOMIC INFORMATION ABOUT AN ENTITY FOR MAKING	· DECISIONS and · INFORMED JUDGMENTS

USERS OF ACCOUNTING INFORMATION

· MANAGEMENT

· INVESTORS

· CREDITORS

· EMPLOYEES

· GOVERNMENTAL AGENCIES

CLASSIFICATIONS OF ACCOUNTING

- FINANCIAL ACCOUNTING

- MANAGERIAL ACCOUNTING / COST ACCOUNTING

- AUDITING - PUBLIC / INTERNAL

- GOVERNMENTAL ACCOUNTING

- INCOME TAX ACCOUNTING

PROFESSIONAL CERTIFICATIONS

- CPA - CERTIFIED PUBLIC ACCOUNTANT

- CMA - CERTIFIED MANAGEMENT ACCOUNTANT

- CIA - CERTIFIED INTERNAL AUDITOR

FINANCIAL ACCOUNTING STANDARD SETTING

FASB (FINANCIAL ACCOUNTING STANDARDS BOARD)

- *STATEMENTS OF FINANCIAL ACCOUNTING STANDARDS* OVER 140 ISSUED. DEAL WITH SPECIFIC ACCOUNTING AND FINANCIAL REPORTING ISSUES.

- *STATEMENTS OF FINANCIAL ACCOUNTING CONCEPTS* 7 ISSUED. AN ATTEMPT TO PROVIDE A COMMON FOUNDATION TO SUPPORT FINANCIAL ACCOUNTING STANDARDS.

- **KEY OBJECTIVES OF FINANCIAL REPORTING (SFAC #1)**

  - RELATE TO EXTERNAL FINANCIAL REPORTING.

  - TO SUPPORT BUSINESS AND ECONOMIC DECISIONS.

  - TO PROVIDE INFORMATION ABOUT CASH FLOWS.

  - PRIMARY FOCUS IS ON EARNINGS BASED ON ACCRUAL ACCOUNTING.

  - NOT TO MEASURE DIRECTLY THE VALUE OF A BUSINESS ENTERPRISE.

  - INFORMATION REPORTED SUBJECT TO EVALUATION BY INDIVIDUAL FINANCIAL STATEMENT USERS.

  - ACCOUNTING STANDARDS ARE STILL EVOLVING.

INTERNATIONAL ACCOUNTING STANDARDS

- IASC (INTERNATIONAL ACCOUNTING STANDARDS COMMITTEE).

- STANDARDS DIFFER SIGNIFICANTLY AMONG COUNTRIES.

- INDIVIDUAL COUNTRY STANDARDS REFLECT LOCAL MARKET NEEDS AND COUNTRY REGULATION AND TAXATION PRACTICES.

ETHICS AND THE ACCOUNTING PROFESSION

- AICPA CODE OF PROFESSIONAL CONDUCT

- IMA STANDARDS OF ETHICAL CONDUCT FOR MANAGEMENT ACCOUNTANTS

KEY ELEMENTS OF ETHICAL BEHAVIOR

- INTEGRITY

- OBJECTIVITY

- INDEPENDENCE

- COMPETENCE

TRANSACTIONS TO FINANCIAL STATEMENTS

	PROCEDURES FOR SORTING, CLASSIFYING AND PRESENTING (BOOKKEEPING)	
TRANSACTIONS →		→ FINANCIAL STATEMENTS
	SELECTION OF ALTERNATIVE METHODS OF REFLECTING THE EFFECTS OF TRANSACTIONS (ACCOUNTING)	

TRANSACTIONS
ECONOMIC INTERCHANGES BETWEEN ENTITIES.

EXAMPLES:

FINANCIAL STATEMENTS
 · **BALANCE SHEET**
   FINANCIAL POSITION AT A POINT IN TIME.

 · **INCOME STATEMENT**
   EARNINGS FOR A PERIOD OF TIME.

 · **STATEMENT OF CASH FLOWS**
   SUMMARY OF CASH FLOWS FOR A PERIOD OF TIME.

 · **STATEMENT OF CHANGES IN OWNERS' EQUITY**
   INVESTMENTS BY OWNERS, EARNINGS OF THE FIRM,
   AND DISTRIBUTIONS TO OWNERS FOR A PERIOD OF TIME.

6

FINANCIAL STATEMENTS

BALANCE SHEET (AT A POINT IN TIME)

EXHIBIT 2-1   Balance Sheet

MAIN STREET STORE, INC.
Balance Sheet
August 31, 2002

Assets		Liabilities and Owners' Equity	
Current assets:		Current liabilities:	
Cash	$ 34,000	Short-term debt	$ 20,000
Accounts receivable	80,000	Accounts payable	35,000
Merchandise inventory	170,000	Other accrued liabilities	12,000
Total current assets	$284,000	Total current	
Plant and equipment:		liabilities	$ 67,000
Equipment	40,000	Long-term debt	50,000
Less: Accumulated		Total liabilities	$117,000
depreciation	(4,000)	Owners' equity	203,000
		Total liabilities and	
Total assets	$320,000	owners' equity	$320,000

KEY RELATIONSHIP

ASSETS = LIABILITIES + OWNERS' EQUITY

KEY TERMINOLOGY

- ASSETS
- CURRENT ASSETS
- ACCUMULATED DEPRECIATION

- LIABILITIES
- CURRENT LIABILITIES
- OWNERS' EQUITY

FINANCIAL STATEMENTS

INCOME STATEMENT (FOR A PERIOD OF TIME)

EXHIBIT 2–2   Income Statement

MAIN STREET STORE, INC.
Income Statement
For the Year Ended August 31, 2002

Net sales	$1,200,000
Cost of goods sold	850,000
Gross profit	$ 350,000
Selling, general, and administrative expenses	311,000
Income from operations	$ 39,000
Interest expense	9,000
Income before taxes	$ 30,000
Income taxes	12,000
Net income	$ 18,000
Net income per share of common stock outstanding	$ 1.80

KEY RELATIONSHIP

REVENUES - EXPENSES = NET INCOME

KEY TERMINOLOGY

- REVENUES (SALES)
- GROSS PROFIT
- EARNINGS BEFORE TAXES
- NET INCOME PER SHARE
  OF COMMON STOCK

- COST OF GOODS SOLD
- OPERATING INCOME
- NET INCOME

8

FINANCIAL STATEMENTS

STATEMENT OF CHANGES IN OWNERS' EQUITY
(FOR A PERIOD OF TIME)

EXHIBIT 2–3 Statement of Changes in Owners' Equity

MAIN STREET STORE, INC.
Statement of Changes in Owners' Equity
For the Year Ended August 31, 2002

Paid-In Capital:		
Beginning balance	$	–0–
Common stock, par value, $10; 50,000 shares authorized;		
10,000 shares issued and outstanding		100,000
Additional paid-in capital		90,000
Balance, August 31, 2002		$190,000
Retained Earnings:		
Beginning balance	$	–0–
Net income for the year		18,000
Less: Cash dividends of $.50 per share		(5,000)
Balance, August 31, 2002		$ 13,000
Total owners' equity		$203,000

TWO PRINCIPAL COMPONENTS

· PAID-IN CAPITAL CHANGES
· RETAINED EARNINGS CHANGES

KEY RELATIONSHIP

   RETAINED EARNINGS BEGINNING BALANCE
 + NET INCOME FOR THE PERIOD
 - DIVIDENDS
 = RETAINED EARNINGS ENDING BALANCE

KEY TERMINOLOGY

· PAID-IN CAPITAL   · DIVIDENDS

FINANCIAL STATEMENTS

STATEMENT OF CASH FLOWS (FOR A PERIOD OF TIME)

EXHIBIT 2—4   Statement of Cash Flows

MAIN STREET STORE, INC.
Statement of Cash Flows
For the Year Ended August 31, 2002

Cash Flows from Operating Activities:	
Net income	$ 18,000
Add (deduct) items not affecting cash:	
Depreciation expense	4,000
Increase in accounts receivable	(80,000)
Increase in merchandise inventory	(170,000)
Increase in current liabilities	67,000
Net cash used by operating activities	$(161,000)
Cash Flows from Investing Activities:	
Cash paid for equipment	$ (40,000)
Cash Flows from Financing Activities:	
Cash received from issue of long-term debt	$ 50,000
Cash received from sale of common stock	190,000
Payment of cash dividend on common stock	(5,000)
Net cash provided by financing activities	$ 235,000
Net increase in cash for the year	$ 34,000

KEY TERMINOLOGY

· CASH FLOWS FROM OPERATING ACTIVITIES

· CASH FLOWS FROM INVESTING ACTIVITIES

· CASH FLOWS FROM FINANCING ACTIVITIES

· CHANGE IN CASH FOR THE YEAR

FINANCIAL STATEMENT RELATIONSHIPS

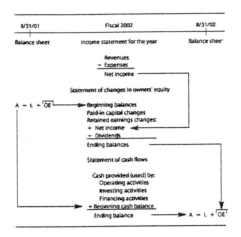

KEY IDEAS

· TRANSACTIONS AFFECTING THE INCOME STATEMENT ALSO AFFECT THE BALANCE SHEET.

· FOR THE BALANCE SHEET TO BALANCE, INCOME STATEMENT

  TRANSACTIONS MUST BE REFLECTED IN THE RETAINED EARNINGS PART OF OWNERS' EQUITY.

· THE STATEMENT OF CASH FLOWS EXPLAINS WHY THE CASH AMOUNT CHANGED DURING THE PERIOD.

11

A MODEL OF THE RELATIONSHIP BETWEEN THE BALANCE SHEET AND INCOME STATEMENT

BALANCE SHEET   INCOME STATEMENT

ASSETS = LIABILITIES + OWNERS' EQUITY ← NET INCOME = REVENUES – EXPENSES

KEY IDEAS

· THE ARROW FROM NET INCOME IN THE INCOME STATEMENT TO OWNERS' EQUITY IN THE BALANCE SHEET INDICATES THAT NET INCOME AFFECTS RETAINED EARNINGS, WHICH IS PART OF OWNERS' EQUITY.

· THE EFFECT OF TRANSACTIONS ON THE FINANCIAL STATEMENTS CAN BE ILLUSTRATED BY ENTERING THE TRANSACTION AMOUNTS IN THE APPROPRIATE COLUMNS.

· THE BALANCE SHEET MUST BE IN BALANCE (A = L + OE) AFTER EVERY TRANSACTION.

ACCOUNTING CONCEPTS AND PRINCIPLES

· ACCOUNTING ENTITY

· ASSETS = LIABILITIES + OWNERS' EQUITY
  (ACCOUNTING EQUATION)

· GOING CONCERN
  (CONTINUITY)

TRANSACTIONS →

PROCEDURES FOR SORTING,
CLASSIFYING AND PRESENTING
(BOOKKEEPING)

SELECTION OF ALTERNATIVE
METHODS OF REFLECTING THE
EFFECTS OF TRANSACTIONS
(ACCOUNTING)

→ FINANCIAL
   STATEMENTS

· UNIT OF
  MEASUREMENT

· COST PRINCIPLE

· OBJECTIVITY

· ACCOUNTING PERIOD

· MATCHING REVENUE
  AND EXPENSE

· REVENUE RECOGNIZED
  AT TIME OF SALE

· ACCRUAL CONCEPT

· CONSISTENCY

· FULL
  DISCLOSURE

· MATERIALITY

· CONSERVATISM

KEY CLARIFICATION

· MATCHING OF REVENUE AND EXPENSE MEANS THAT ALL
  EXPENSES INCURRED IN GENERATING REVENUES FOR
  THE PERIOD ARE SUBTRACTED FROM THOSE REVENUES
  TO DETERMINE NET INCOME. MATCHING DOES <u>NOT</u>
  MEAN THAT REVENUES EQUAL EXPENSES.

13

MEASUREMENTS AND TREND ANALYSIS

- PAT'S GPA LAST SEMESTER: **2.8**

  <u>JUDGMENT:</u> SO WHAT? HOW WELL HAS PAT PERFORMED?

- PAT'S GPA FOR THE LAST FOUR SEMESTERS: **1.9, 2.3, 2.6, 2.8**

  <u>JUDGMENT:</u> PAT'S PERFORMANCE HAS BEEN IMPROVING.

- GPA FOR ALL STUDENTS FOR LAST FOUR SEMESTERS: **2.85, 2.76, 2.70, 2.65**

  <u>JUDGMENT:</u> PAT'S PERFORMANCE HAS IMPROVED WHILE THE PERFORMANCE OF ALL STUDENTS HAS DECLINED.

<u>KEY POINTS</u>

- THE TREND OF DATA IS FREQUENTLY MORE SIGNIFICANT THAN THE DATA ITSELF.

- COMPARISON OF INDIVIDUAL AND GROUP TRENDS IS IMPORTANT WHEN MAKING JUDGMENTS.

RETURN ON INVESTMENT

RATE OF RETURN (**ROI**)

$$\text{RATE OF RETURN} = \frac{\text{AMOUNT OF RETURN}}{\text{AMOUNT INVESTED}}$$

KEY POINTS

· RATE OF RETURN IS AN ANNUAL PERCENTAGE RATE UNLESS OTHERWISE SPECIFIED, THEREFORE

· THE AMOUNT OF RETURN IS THE AMOUNT RECEIVED DURING THE YEAR, (i.e., **NET INCOME** FROM THE INCOME STATEMENT), AND

· THE AMOUNT INVESTED IS THE AVERAGE AMOUNT INVESTED DURING THE YEAR (i.e., **AVERAGE TOTAL ASSETS** FROM THE BALANCE SHEET).

· **ROI IS A SIGNIFICANT MEASURE OF ECONOMIC PERFORMANCE BECAUSE IT DESCRIBES THE RESULTS OBTAINED BY MANAGEMENT'S USE OF THE ASSETS MADE AVAILABLE FOR INVESTMENT DURING THE YEAR.**

THE DUPONT MODEL FOR CALCULATING ROI

$$ROI = MARGIN * TURNOVER$$

$$= \frac{NET\ INCOME}{SALES} * \frac{SALES}{AVERAGE\ TOTAL\ ASSETS}$$

KEY IDEAS

- MARGIN DESCRIBES THE PROFITABILITY FROM SALES.

- TURNOVER DESCRIBES THE EFFICIENCY WITH WHICH ASSETS HAVE BEEN USED TO GENERATE SALES.

- OVERALL PROFITABILITY - RETURN ON INVESTMENT - IS A FUNCTION OF BOTH PROFITABILITY OF SALES AND THE EFFICIENT USE OF ASSETS.

KEY POINTS

- NET INCOME AND SALES ARE FOR THE YEAR. FOR CONSISTENCY, TOTAL ASSETS IS THE AVERAGE OF TOTAL ASSETS FROM THE BALANCE SHEETS AT THE BEGINNING AND END OF THE YEAR.

- OPERATING INCOME MAY BE USED IN THE MARGIN CALCULATION INSTEAD OF NET INCOME, AND AVERAGE OPERATING ASSETS MAY BE USED IN THE TURNOVER CALCULATION. AS LONG AS THE DATA USED ARE CONSISTENTLY CALCULATED, THE TREND OF ROI WILL BE USEFUL FOR JUDGMENTS.

16

RETURN ON EQUITY (ROE)

RETURN ON EQUITY = $\dfrac{\text{NET INCOME}}{\text{AVERAGE OWNERS' EQUITY}}$

KEY POINT

- AS IN ROI, NET INCOME IS <u>FOR THE YEAR</u>, THEREFORE IT IS RELATED TO THE AVERAGE OF THE OWNERS' EQUITY AT THE BEGINNING AND END OF THE YEAR.

KEY IDEAS

- ROI RELATES NET INCOME TO AVERAGE TOTAL ASSETS, AND EXPRESSES A RATE OF RETURN ON THE ASSETS USED BY THE FIRM.

- ROE RELATES NET INCOME TO AVERAGE OWNERS' EQUITY, AND EXPRESSES A RATE OF RETURN ON THAT PORTION OF THE ASSETS PROVIDED BY THE OWNERS OF THE FIRM.

WORKING CAPITAL AND MEASURES OF LIQUIDITY

WORKING CAPITAL

```
    CURRENT ASSETS
  - CURRENT LIABILITIES
  = WORKING CAPITAL
```

KEY DEFINITIONS

· CURRENT ASSETS: CASH AND ASSETS LIKELY TO BE CONVERTED TO CASH WITHIN A YEAR.

· CURRENT LIABILITIES: OBLIGATIONS THAT MUST BE PAID WITHIN A YEAR.

KEY IDEA

· A MEASURE OF THE FIRM'S ABILITY TO PAY ITS CURRENT OBLIGATIONS.

CURRENT RATIO

$$\frac{\text{CURRENT ASSETS}}{\text{CURRENT LIABILITIES}} = \text{CURRENT RATIO}$$

KEY IDEA

· THE CURRENT RATIO IS USUALLY A MORE USEFUL MEASUREMENT THAN THE AMOUNT OF WORKING CAPITAL BECAUSE IT IS A RATIO MEASUREMENT.

WORKING CAPITAL AND MEASURES OF LIQUIDITY

ACID-TEST RATIO (sometimes called QUICK RATIO)

$$\frac{\text{CASH (INCLUDING TEMPORARY CASH INVESTMENTS) + ACCOUNTS RECEIVABLE}}{\text{CURRENT LIABILITIES}}$$

KEY IDEAS

- BY FOCUSING ON CASH AND ACCOUNTS RECEIVABLE, THE ACID-TEST RATIO PROVIDES A MORE SHORT-TERM MEASURE OF LIQUIDITY THAN THE CURRENT RATIO.

- THE ACID-TEST RATIO EXCLUDES INVENTORY, PREPAID EXPENSES, AND OTHER CURRENT ASSETS FROM THE NUMERATOR.

VERTICAL GRAPH SCALES

ARITHMETIC SCALE

KEY FEATURE

- VERTICAL SCALE DISTANCES ARE EQUAL.

KEY IDEA

- A CONSTANT RATE OF GROWTH PLOTS AS AN INCREASINGLY STEEP LINE OVER TIME.

LOGARITHMIC SCALE

KEY FEATURE

- VERTICAL SCALE DISTANCES ARE INCREASINGLY NARROW AND COMPRESSED.

KEY IDEA

- A CONSTANT RATE OF GROWTH PLOTS AS A STRAIGHT LINE.

KEY OBSERVATIONS

- THE HORIZONTAL SCALE WILL ALMOST ALWAYS BE AN ARITHMETIC SCALE, WITH EQUAL DISTANCE BETWEEN THE DATES OF DATA OBSERVATIONS.

- SEMI-LOGARITHMIC FORMAT MEANS THAT THE ONLY THE VERTICAL SCALE IS LOGARITHMIC; THE HORIZONTAL SCALE IS ARITHMETIC.

ARITHMETIC AND SEMI-LOGARITHMIC PLOTS

ARITHMETIC PLOT

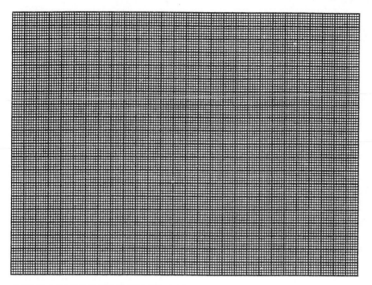

SEMI-LOGARITHMIC PLOT

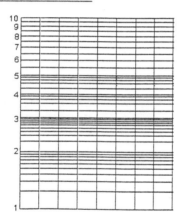

TRANSACTIONS AND THE FINANCIAL STATEMENTS

KEY IDEAS

- TRANSACTIONS AFFECT THE BALANCE SHEET AND/OR THE INCOME STATEMENT.

- THE BALANCE SHEET MUST BE IN BALANCE AFTER EVERY TRANSACTION.

- THE RETAINED EARNINGS ACCOUNT ON THE BALANCE SHEET INCLUDES NET INCOME FROM THE INCOME STATEMENT.

- BALANCE SHEET ACCOUNTS MAY HAVE BALANCES AT THE END OF A FISCAL PERIOD, AND BEFORE TRANSACTIONS OF THE SUBSEQUENT PERIOD ARE RECORDED.

KEY TERMINOLOGY

- EACH INDIVIDUAL ASSET, LIABILITY, OWNERS' EQUITY, REVENUE, OR EXPENSE "ACCOUNT" MAY ADDITIONALLY BE DESCRIBED WITH ITS CATEGORY TITLE. EXAMPLES:
    - "CASH ASSET ACCOUNT"
    - "ACCOUNTS PAYABLE LIABILITY ACCOUNT"
    - "COMMON STOCK OWNERS' EQUITY ACCOUNT"
    - "SALES REVENUE ACCOUNT"
    - "WAGES EXPENSE ACCOUNT"

KEY RELATIONSHIP

- TRANSACTIONS DURING A FISCAL PERIOD CAUSE THE BALANCE OF THE AFFECTED ACCOUNT(S) TO INCREASE OR DECREASE. BOOKKEEPING IS THE POCESS OF KEEPING TRACK OF THESE CHANGES.

BOOKKEEPING PROCEDURES

WHAT THE BOOKS ARE CALLED

- THE **JOURNAL** IS A CHRONOLOGICAL RECORD OF EACH TRANSACTION.

- THE **LEDGER** IS A BOOK OF ALL OF THE ACCOUNTS; ACCOUNTS ARE USUALLY ARRANGED IN THE SEQUENCE FOUND ON THE BALANCE SHEET AND INCOME STATEMENT, RESPECTIVELY.

HOW TRANSACTIONS ARE RECORDED

- ACCOUNTS ARE FREQUENTLY IN THE SHAPE OF A T

- THE LEFT-HAND SIDE OF THE "T ACCOUNT" IS CALLED THE **DEBIT** SIDE.

- THE RIGHT-HAND SIDE OF THE "T ACCOUNT" IS CALLED THE **CREDIT** SIDE.

- AN INCREASE IN AN ASSET OR AN EXPENSE ACCOUNT IS RECORDED AS A DEBIT; A DECREASE IN EITHER AN ASSET OR AN EXPENSE ACCOUNT IS RECORDED AS A CREDIT.

- AN INCREASE IN A LIABILITY, OWNERS' EQUITY OR REVENUE ACCOUNT IS RECORDED AS A CREDIT; A DECREASE IN EITHER A LIABILITY, OWNERS' EQUITY, OR REVENUE ACCOUNT IS RECORDED AS A DEBIT.

BOOKKEEPING PROCEDURES

- A TRANSACTION IS INITIALLY RECORDED IN A JOURNAL ENTRY.

- THE JOURNAL ENTRY IS THEN **POSTED** TO THE LEDGER ACCOUNTS THAT HAVE BEEN AFFECTED BY THE TRANSACTION.

KEY IDEAS

- A TRANSACTION WILL AFFECT AT LEAST TWO ACCOUNTS, AND CAN AFFECT MANY ACCOUNTS.

- BECAUSE THE BALANCE SHEET MUST BALANCE AFTER EVERY TRANSACTION, THE DEBIT(S) AND CREDIT(S) AMOUNTS OF EACH JOURNAL ENTRY MUST BE EQUAL.

DEBITS = CREDITS

KEY OBSERVATION

- EACH ACCOUNT HAS A **"NORMAL BALANCE"** SIDE - DEBIT OR CREDIT - THAT IS CONSISTENT WITH THE KIND OF ENTRY THAT CAUSES THE ACCOUNT BALANCE TO **INCREASE**.

DEBIT	**CREDIT**
ASSETS	LIABILITIES
EXPENSES	OWNERS' EQUITY
	REVENUES

TRANSACTION ANALYSIS METHODOLOGY

FIVE QUESTIONS OF TRANSACTION ANALYSIS

KEY IDEA

· TO UNDERSTAND EITHER THE BOOKKEEPING
   PROCEDURE FOR A TRANSACTION, OR THE EFFECT
   OF A TRANSACTION ON THE FINANCIAL STATEMENTS,
   THE FOLLOWING QUESTIONS MUST BE ANSWERED:

   1. WHAT'S GOING ON?
      (WHAT IS THE NATURE OF THE TRANSACTION?)

   2. WHAT ACCOUNTS ARE AFFECTED?
      (WHAT IS THE FINANCIAL STATEMENT CATEGORY
      OF EACH ACCOUNT - ASSET, LIABILITY, OWNERS'
      EQUITY, REVENUE OR EXPENSE?)

   3. HOW IS EACH ACCOUNT AFFECTED?
      (IS THE BALANCE INCREASING OR DECREASING?)

   4. DOES THE BALANCE SHEET BALANCE?
      (DO THE DEBITS EQUAL THE CREDITS? IS THE
      BALANCE SHEET EQUATION STILL IN BALANCE
      AFTER RECORDING THE TRANSACTION?)

   > **DEBITS = CREDITS?**
   >
   > **ASSETS = LIABLIITIES + OWNERS' EQUITY?**

   5. DOES MY ANALYSIS MAKE SENSE?
      (DO THE ACCOUNT BALANCES OR THE FINANCIAL
      STATEMENTS REFLECT THE EFFECT OF THE
      TRANSACTION?)

25

AN ALTERNATIVE TO DEBIT AND CREDIT BOOKKEEPING

THE FINANCIAL STATEMENT RELATIONSHIP MODEL

BALANCE SHEET	INCOME STATEMENT
ASSETS = LIABILITIES + OWNERS' EQUITY ← NET INCOME = REVENUES – EXPENSES	

KEY POINTS

· SHOW THE EFFECT OF EACH TRANSACTION IN THE APPROPRIATE COLUMN OF THE MODEL. SHOW ACCOUNT NAMES FOR ADDITIONAL PRECISION.

· BECAUSE NET INCOME INCREASES OWNERS' EQUITY, INCREASES IN REVENUES APPEAR AS POSITIVE AMOUNTS, AND INCREASES IN EXPENSES (WHICH DECREASE NET INCOME) APPEAR AS NEGATIVE AMOUNTS.

· KEEP THE EQUATION IN BALANCE FOR EACH TRANSACTION BY ENTERING (OR VISUALIZING) AN EQUAL SIGN BETWEEN ASSETS AND LIABILITIES.

KEY IDEA

· USE OF THIS MODEL FOCUSES ON THE IMPACT OF TRANSACTIONS ON THE FINANCIAL STATEMENTS WITHOUT CONCERN FOR BOOKKEEPING JARGON.

ADJUSTING ENTRIES

<u>WHAT ARE THEY? WHY DO THEM?</u>

- ADJUSTING ENTRIES, OR ADJUSTMENTS, ARE "UPDATES" AND "CORRECTIONS" MADE TO INCREASE THE ACCURACY OF THE INFORMATION IN THE FINANCIAL STATEMENTS.

- **RECLASSIFICATIONS:**
  THE BOOKKEEPING FOR THE ORIGINAL TRANSACTION WAS APPROPRIATE WHEN IT WAS RECORDED, BUT THE PASSAGE OF TIME REQUIRES A RECLASSIFICATION OF THE ORIGINAL BOOKKEEPING TO REFLECT CORRECT ACCOUNT BALANCES AS OF THE DATE OF THE FINANCIAL STATEMENTS.

- **ACCRUALS:**
  REVENUES WERE EARNED OR EXPENSES WERE INCURRED DURING THE PERIOD, BUT NO TRANSACTION WAS RECORDED, (BECAUSE NO CASH WAS RECEIVED OR PAID). THEREFORE, IT IS NECESSARY TO **ACCRUE** THE EFFECT OF THE TRANSACTION AS OF THE DATE OF THE FINANCIAL STATEMENTS.

<u>KEY IDEAS</u>

- ACCRUAL ACCOUNTING MEANS THAT REVENUES ARE RECOGNIZED WHEN <u>EARNED</u> (NOT WHEN CASH IS RECEIVED) AND THAT EXPENSES ARE REFLECTED IN THE PERIOD IN WHICH THEY ARE <u>INCURRED</u> (NOT WHEN CASH IS PAID).

- ADJUSTING ENTRIES RESULT IN MATCHING REVENUES AND EXPENSES, WHICH IS THE OBJECTIVE OF ACCRUAL ACCOUNTING.

CURRENT ASSETS

DEFINITION

- CURRENT ASSETS ARE CASH AND THOSE ASSETS EXPECTED TO BE CONVERTED TO CASH OR USED UP IN THE OPERATING ACTIVITIES OF THE ENTITY WITHIN ONE YEAR.

ACCOUNTS THAT COMPRISE CURRENT ASSETS

- CASH

- MARKETABLE (OR SHORT-TERM) SECURITIES

- ACCOUNTS AND NOTES RECEIVABLE

- INVENTORIES

- PREPAID EXPENSES

KEY IDEA

- EVERY ENTITY HAS AN OPERATING CYCLE IN WHICH PRODUCTS AND SERVICES ARE PURCHASED, SERVICES ARE PERFORMED ON ACCOUNT (USUALLY), PAYMENT IS MADE TO EMPLOYEES AND SUPPLIERS, AND FINALLY CASH IS RECEIVED FROM CUSTOMERS. IF THE ENTITY IS A MANUFACTURER, PRODUCT IS MADE AND HELD AS INVENTORY BEFORE IT IS SOLD. CURRENT ASSETS REFLECT THE INVESTMENT REQUIRED TO SUPPORT THIS CYCLE.

CASH AND MARKETABLE SECURITIES

<u>KEY IDEAS</u>

- THE CASH AMOUNT ON THE BALANCE SHEET IS THE AMOUNT OF CASH OWNED BY THE ENTITY ON THE BALANCE SHEET DATE.

    - THUS THE LEDGER ACCOUNT BALANCE OF CASH MUST BE RECONCILED WITH THE BANK STATEMENT ENDING BALANCE, AND THE LEDGER ACCOUNT BALANCE MUST BE ADJUSTED AS NECESSARY.

    - THE ADJUSTMENT WILL REFLECT BANK TIMING DIFFERENCES AND BOOK ERRORS.

- SHORT-TERM MARKETABLE SECURITIES THAT WILL BE HELD UNTIL MATURITY ARE SHOWN ON THE BALANCE SHEET AT COST, WHICH IS USUALLY ABOUT THE SAME AS MARKET VALUE.

- SECURITIES EXPECTED TO BE HELD FOR SEVERAL MONTHS AFTER THE BALANCE SHEET DATE ARE SHOWN AT THEIR MARKET VALUE.

- INTEREST INCOME FROM MARKETABLE SECURITIES THAT HAS NOT BEEN RECEIVED MUST BE ACCRUED.

ACCOUNTS RECEIVABLE

KEY ISSUES

- ACCOUNTS RECEIVABLE ARE REPORTED ON THE BALANCE SHEET AT THEIR "NET REALIZABLE VALUE," WHICH IS THE AMOUNT OF CASH EXPECTED TO BE COLLECTED FROM THE ACCOUNTS RECEIVABLE.

- WHEN SALES ARE MADE ON ACCOUNT, THERE IS A VERY HIGH PROBABILITY THAT SOME ACCOUNTS RECEIVABLE WILL NOT BE COLLECTED.

- THE MATCHING OF REVENUES AND EXPENSES CONCEPT REQUIRES THAT THE "COST" OF UNCOLLECTIBLE ACCOUNTS RECEIVABLE BE REPORTED IN THE SAME PERIOD AS THE REVENUE THAT WAS RECOGNIZED WHEN THE ACCOUNT RECEIVABLE WAS CREATED.

KEY POINTS

- THE "COST" OF UNCOLLECTIBLE ACCOUNTS (BAD DEBTS EXPENSE) MUST BE ESTIMATED. THIS LEADS TO A VALUATION ADJUSTMENT.

- THE AMOUNT OF ACCOUNTS RECEIVABLE NOT EXPECTED TO BE COLLECTED IS RECORDED AND REPORTED IN AN "ALLOWANCE FOR BAD DEBTS" ACOUNT.

- THE ALLOWANCE FOR BAD DEBTS ACCOUNT IS A "CONTRA ASSET" REPORTED IN THE BALANCE SHEET AS A SUBTRACTION FROM ACCOUNTS RECEIVABLE.

INTERNAL CONTROL STRUCTURE

KEY IDEA

- THE ENTITY NEEDS TO HAVE ADMINISTRATIVE CONTROLS AND ACCOUNTING CONTROLS TO SUPPORT ACHIEVEMENT OF ORGANIZATIONAL GOALS AND SOUND ACCOUNTING AND FINANCIAL REPORTING PROCEDURES.

ACCOUNTING CONTROLS

- ASSURE ACCURACY OF BOOKKEEPING RECORDS AND FINANCIAL STATEMENTS.

- PROTECT ASSETS FROM UNAUTHORIZED USE OR LOSS.

ADMINISTRATIVE CONTROLS

- ENCOURAGE ADHERENCE TO MANAGEMENT'S POLICIES.

- PROVIDE FOR EFFICIENT OPERATIONS.

KEY OBSERVATION

- INTERNAL CONTROLS ARE POSITIVE; THEY SUPPORT ACHIEVEMENT OF ORGANIZATIONAL OBJECTIVES.

INVENTORIES

<u>WHAT'S GOING ON?</u>

- THE INVENTORY ASSET ACCOUNT CONTAINS THE COST OF ITEMS THAT ARE BEING HELD FOR SALE. WHEN AN ITEM OF INVENTORY IS SOLD, ITS COST IS TRANSFERRED FROM THE INVENTORY ASSET ACCOUNT (IN THE BALANCE SHEET) TO THE COST OF GOODS SOLD EXPENSE ACCOUNT (IN THE INCOME STATEMENT).

- THIS IS A TRANSACTION SEPARATE FROM THE SALE TRANSACTION, WHICH RESULTS IN AN INCREASE IN AN ASSET ACCOUNT IN THE BALANCE SHEET (EITHER ACCOUNTS RECEIVABLE OR CASH), AND AN INCREASE IN SALES, A REVENUE ACCOUNT IN THE INCOME STATEMENT.

<u>KEY ISSUE</u>

- WHEN THE INVENTORY INCLUDES THE COST OF SEVERAL UNITS OF THE ITEM SOLD, HOW IS THE COST OF THE ITEM SOLD DETERMINED?

INVENTORY COST FLOW ASSUMPTIONS

ALTERNATIVE COST FLOW ASSUMPTIONS

- SPECIFIC IDENTIFICATION

- WEIGHTED AVERAGE

- FIFO - **F**IRST COST **I**N TO INVENTORY,
     FIRST COST **O**UT TO COST OF GOODS SOLD

- LIFO - **L**AST COST **I**N TO INVENTORY,
     FIRST COST **O**UT TO COST OF GOODS SOLD

KEY ISSUES

- HOW DO CHANGES IN THE <u>COST</u> OF INVENTORY
  ITEMS OVER TIME AFFECT COST OF GOODS SOLD
  UNDER EACH OF THE COST FLOW ASSUMPTIONS?

- HOW DO CHANGES IN THE <u>QUANTITY</u> OF INVENTORY
  ITEMS AFFECT COST OF GOODS SOLD UNDER
  EACH OF THE COST FLOW ASSUMPTIONS?

KEY POINT

- ROI, ROE, AND MEASURES OF LIQUIDITY WILL BE
  AFFECTED BY THE INVENTORY COST FLOW
  ASSUMPTION USED WHEN THE COST OF
  INVENTORY ITEMS CHANGES OVER TIME.

PREPAID EXPENSES

<u>WHAT'S GOING ON?</u>

· PREPAID EXPENSES RESULT FROM THE
APPLICATION OF ACCRUAL ACCOUNTING.
SOME EXPENDITURES MADE IN ONE PERIOD ARE
NOT PROPERLY RECOGNIZABLE AS EXPENSES UNTIL
A SUBSEQUENT PERIOD.

· IN THESE SITUATIONS, EXPENSE RECOGNITION IS
DEFERRED UNTIL THE PERIOD IN WHICH THE
EXENSE APPLIES.

<u>PREPAID EXPENSES FREQUENTLY INCLUDE:</u>

· INSURANCE PREMIUMS

· RENT

NONCURRENT ASSETS

<u>KEY TERMINOLOGY</u>

· DEPRECIATION EXPENSE / ACCUMULATED DEPRECIATION

DEPRECIATION EXPENSE REFERS TO THAT PORTION OF THE COST OF A LONG-LIVED ASSET RECORDED AS AN EXPENSE IN AN ACCOUNTING PERIOD. DEPRECIATION IN ACCOUNTING IS THE SPREADING OF THE COST OF A NONCURRENT ASSET OVER ITS ESTIMATED USEFUL LIFE TO THE ENTITY. THIS IS AN APPLICATION OF THE MATCHING CONCEPT.

ACCUMULATED DEPRECIATION IS A CONTRA ASSET ACCOUNT. THE BALANCE IN THIS ACCOUNT IS THE ACCUMULATED TOTAL OF ALL OF THE DEPRECIATION EXPENSE RECOGNIZED TO DATE ON THE RELATED ASSET(S).

· CAPITALIZE / EXPENSE

TO **CAPITALIZE** AN EXPENDITURE MEANS TO RECORD THE EXPENDITURE AS AN ASSET. A NONCURRENT ASSET THAT HAS BEEN CAPITALIZED WILL BE DEPRECIATED.

TO **EXPENSE** AN EXPENDITURE MEANS TO RECORD THE EXPENDITURE AS AN EXPENSE.

· NET BOOK VALUE

THE DIFFERENCE BETWEEN AN ASSET'S COST AND ITS ACCUMULATED DEPRECIATION IS ITS **NET BOOK VALUE**.

DEPRECIATION OF NONCURRENT ASSETS

KEY POINT

· THE RECOGNITION OF DEPRECIATION EXPENSE
  DOES NOT AFFECT CASH.

DEPRECIATION EXPENSE CALCULATION ELEMENTS

· ASSET COST

· ESTIMATED SALVAGE VALUE

· ESTIMATED USEFUL LIFE TO ENTITY

ALTERNATIVE CALCULATION METHODS

· STRAIGHT-LINE
    · BASED ON YEARS OF LIFE
    · BASED ON UNITS OF PRODUCTION

· ACCELERATED
    · SUM-OF-THE-YEARS-DIGITS
    · DECLINING-BALANCE

DEPRECIATION METHOD ALTERNATIVES

<u>KEY POINTS</u>

· ACCELERATED DEPRECIATION RESULTS IN GREATER DEPRECIATION EXPENSE DURING THE EARLY YEARS OF THE ASSET'S LIFE THAN STRAIGHT-LINE DEPRECIATION. MOST FIRMS USE STRAIGHT-LINE DEPRECIATION FOR FINANCIAL REPORTING PURPOSES.

· DEPRECIATION EXPENSE DOES NOT AFFECT CASH, BUT BECAUSE DEPRECIATION IS DEDUCTIBLE FOR INCOME TAX PURPOSES, MOST FIRMS USE AN ACCELERATED METHOD FOR CALCULATING INCOME TAX DEPRECIATION.

· THE DEPRECIATION METHOD SELECTED FOR FINANCIAL REPORTING PURPOSES WILL HAVE AN EFFECT ON ROI AND ROE. TO MAKE VALID COMPARISONS BETWEEN COMPANIES, IT IS NECESSARY TO KNOW WHETHER OR NOT COMPARABLE DEPRECIATION CALCULATION METHODS HAVE BEEN USED.

· IF AN EXPENDITURE HAS BEEN INAPPROPRIATELY CAPITALIZED OR EXPENSED, BOTH ASSETS AND NET INCOME WILL BE AFFECTED, IN THE CURRENT YEAR AND IN FUTURE YEARS OF THE ASSET'S LIFE.

ASSETS ACQUIRED BY CAPITAL LEASE

KEY IDEAS

- A LONG-TERM LEASE IS FREQUENTLY A WAY OF FINANCING THE ACQUISITION OF A NONCURRENT ASSET.

- THE EFFECT OF THE ACCOUNTING FOR A LEASED ASSET SHOULD NOT BE DIFFERENT FROM THE ACCOUNTING FOR A PURCHASED ASSET.

ACCOUNTING FOR A LEASED ASSET

- THE "COST" OF A LEASED ASSET IS THE PRESENT VALUE OF THE LEASE OBLIGATIONS.

- DEPRECIATION EXPENSE IS RECORDED BASED ON THIS "COST".

- AS ANNUAL LEASE PAYMENTS ARE MADE, INTEREST EXPENSE IS RECOGNIZED AND THE LEASE OBLIGATION IS REDUCED.

INTANGIBLE ASSETS AND NATURAL RESOURCES

KEY POINT

- ALTHOUGH THE TERMINOLOGY IS DIFFERENT
  FROM THAT USED FOR DEPRECIABLE ASSETS, THE
  ACCOUNTING IS ESSENTIALLY THE SAME: THE
  EXPENDITURE IS CAPITALIZED, AND THE EXPENSE
  IS RECOGNIZED PERIODICALLY OVER THE USEFUL
  LIFE OF THE ASSET TO THE ENTITY.

TERMINOLOGY

- **INTANGIBLE ASSETS**

    AMORTIZATION EXPENSE

    USUALLY AN ACCUMULATED AMORTIZATION
    ACCOUNT IS NOT USED.

- **NATURAL RESOURCES**

    DEPLETION EXPENSE

    ACCUMULATED DEPLETION

PRESENT VALUE ANALYSIS

<u>KEY IDEAS</u>

· MONEY HAS VALUE OVER TIME.

· AN AMOUNT TO BE RECEIVED OR PAID IN THE
  FUTURE HAS A VALUE TODAY (PRESENT VALUE)
  THAT IS LESS THAN THE FUTURE VALUE.

  WHY? BECAUSE OF THE INTEREST THAT CAN BE
  EARNED BETWEEN THE PRESENT AND THE FUTURE.

<u>KEY RELATIONSHIP</u>

· A TIME LINE APPROACH CREATES A VISUAL IMAGE
  THAT MAKES THE TIME VALUE OF MONEY CONCEPT
  EASY TO WORK WITH.

  WHAT IS THE PRESENT VALUE OF $ 4,000 TO BE
  RECEIVED OR PAID IN 4 YEARS, AT AN INTEREST
  RATE OF 8%?

		Interest Rate = 8%		
TODAY	1	2	3	4

AMOUNT DUE IN 4 YEARS $ 4,000
PRESENT VALUE FACTOR (TABLE 6-2)   * .7350

$2,940

THE VALUE TODAY OF $4,000 TO BE PAID OR RECEIVED
IN 4 YEARS, ASSUMING AN INTEREST RATE OF 8%, IS
$2,940.

CURRENT LIABILITIES

DEFINITION

- CURRENT LIABILITIES ARE THOSE THAT MUST BE
  PAID WITHIN ONE YEAR OF THE BALANCE SHEET DATE.

ACCOUNTS THAT COMPRISE CURRENT LIABILITIES

- SHORT-TERM DEBT

- ACCOUNTS PAYABLE

- VARIOUS ACCRUED LIABILITIES, INCLUDING:

  - WAGES   · OPERATING EXPENSES
  - INTEREST   · TAXES

- CURRENT MATURITIES OF LONG-TERM DEBT

KEY IDEAS

- A PRINCIPAL CONCERN ABOUT LIABILITIES IS THAT
  THEY ARE NOT UNDERSTATED. IF LIABILITIES ARE TOO
  LOW, EXPENSES ARE PROBABLY UNDERSTATED ALSO,
  WHICH MEANS THAT NET INCOME IS OVERSTATED.

- THE AMOUNT OF CURRENT LIABILITIES IS RELATED
  TO THE AMOUNT OF CURRENT ASSETS TO MEASURE
  THE FIRM'S **LIQUIDITY** -- ITS ABILITY TO PAY ITS BILLS
  WHEN THEY COME DUE.

INTEREST CALCULATION METHODS

BASIC MODEL FOR CALCULATING INTEREST

INTEREST = **PRINCIPAL** * ANNUAL **RATE** * **TIME** IN YEARS

KEY ISSUE

- IS THE PRINCIPAL AMOUNT USED IN THE INTEREST CALCULATION EQUAL TO THE CASH ACTUALLY AVAILABLE FOR THE BORROWER TO USE?

STRAIGHT INTEREST

- PRINCIPAL USED IN THE INTEREST CALCULATION IS EQUAL TO THE CASH RECEIVED BY THE BORROWER.

- INTEREST IS PAID TO THE LENDER PERIODICALLY DURING THE TERM OF THE LOAN, OR AT THE LOAN MATURITY DATE.

DISCOUNT

- PRINCIPAL USED IN THE INTEREST CALCULATION IS THE "AMOUNT BORROWED", BUT THEN INTEREST IS SUBTRACTED FROM THAT PRINCIPAL TO GET THE AMOUNT OF CASH MADE AVAILABLE TO THE BORROWER. THIS RESULTS IN AN EFFECTIVE INTEREST RATE (APR) GREATER THAN THE RATE USED IN THE INTEREST CALCULATION.

- BECAUSE INTEREST WAS PAID IN ADVANCE, ONLY THE PRINCIPAL AMOUNT IS REPAID AT THE LOAN MATURITY DATE.

FINANCIAL LEVERAGE

<u>KEY IDEAS</u>

- WHEN MONEY IS BORROWED AT A FIXED INTEREST
  RATE, THE DIFFERENCE BETWEEN THE ROI EARNED
  ON THAT MONEY AND THE INTEREST RATE PAID
  AFFECTS THE WEALTH OF THE BORROWER. THIS
  IS CALLED FINANCIAL LEVERAGE.

- FINANCIAL LEVERAGE IS POSITIVE WHEN THE ROI
  EARNED ON BORROWED MONEY IS GREATER THAN
  THE INTEREST RATE PAID ON THE BORROWED MONEY.
  FINANCIAL LEVERAGE IS NEGATIVE WHEN THE
  OPPOSITE OCCURS.

- FINANCIAL LEVERAGE INCREASES THE RISK THAT A
  FIRM'S ROI WILL FLUCTUATE, BECAUSE ROI CHANGES
  AS BUSINESS CONDITIONS AND THE FIRM'S OPERATING
  RESULTS CHANGE, BUT THE INTEREST RATE ON
  BORROWED FUNDS IS USUALLY FIXED.

LONG-TERM DEBT (BONDS PAYABLE)

<u>KEY IDEA</u>

· FIRMS ISSUE LONG-TERM DEBT (BONDS PAYABLE)
TO GET SOME OF THE FUNDS NEEDED TO INVEST IN
ASSETS. THE OWNERS DO NOT USUALLY PROVIDE ALL
OF THE NECESSARY FUNDS BECAUSE IT IS USUALLY
DESIRABLE TO HAVE SOME FINANCIAL LEVERAGE.

<u>BOND CHARACTERISTICS</u>

· A FIXED INTEREST RATE (USUALLY) CALLED THE
STATED RATE OR **COUPON** RATE.

> · INTEREST USUALLY PAYABLE SEMI-ANNUALLY.

> · INDIVIDUAL BONDS USUALLY HAVE A FACE
> AMOUNT (PRINCIPAL) OF $1,000.

> · BOND PRICES ARE STATED AS A % OF THE FACE
> AMOUNT; FOR EXAMPLE, A PRICE QUOTE OF 98.3
> MEANS 98.3% OF $1000, OR $983.

> · MOST BONDS HAVE A STATED MATURITY DATE -
> BUT MOST BONDS ARE ALSO **CALLABLE**; THEY CAN
> BE REDEEMED PRIOR TO MATURITY AT THE OPTION
> OF THE ISSUER.

> · FREQUENTLY SOME COLLATERAL IS PROVIDED BY
> THE ISSUER.

BOND MARKET VALUE

KEY POINT

· THE MARKET VALUE OF A BOND IS A FUNCTION OF
  THE RELATIONSHIP BETWEEN MARKET INTEREST
  RATES AND THE BOND'S STATED OR COUPON
  RATE OF INTEREST.

  · AS MARKET INTEREST RATES FALL, THE MARKET
    VALUE OF A BOND RISES.

  · AS MARKET INTEREST RATES RISE, THE MARKET
    VALUE OF A BOND FALLS.

WHAT'S GOING ON?

· A BOND'S STATED OR COUPON RATE OF INTEREST IS
  FIXED AND STAYS THE SAME REGARDLESS OF WHAT
  HAPPENS TO MARKET INTEREST RATES.   THEREFORE,
  IF MARKET INTEREST RATES RISE ABOVE THE STATED
  OR COUPON RATE, THE BOND BECOMES LESS VALUABLE
  TO INVESTORS.

KEY RELATIONSHIP

· THE MARKET VALUE OF A BOND IS THE PRESENT
  VALUE OF THE FUTURE PAYMENTS OF INTEREST AND
  PRINCIPAL, BASED ON (i.e., DISCOUNTED AT) MARKET
  INTEREST RATES.

45

BOND PREMIUM AND DISCOUNT

KEY IDEA

- WHEN THE MARKET INTEREST RATE AT THE
  DATE A BOND IS ISSUED IS DIFFERENT FROM
  THE STATED OR COUPON RATE OF THE BOND,
  THE BOND WILL BE ISSUED AT:

  - A PREMIUM (MARKET INTEREST RATE <
    STATED OR COUPON RATE)

  - OR A DISCOUNT (MARKET INTEREST RATE >
    STATED OR COUPON RATE).

KEY POINTS

- WHEN A BOND IS ISSUED AT A PREMIUM, THE
  PREMIUM IS AMORTIZED TO INTEREST EXPENSE
  OVER THE TERM OF THE BOND, RESULTING IN
  LOWER ANNUAL INTEREST EXPENSE THAN
  THE INTEREST PAID ON THE BOND.

- WHEN A BOND IS ISSUED AT A DISCOUNT, THE
  DISCOUNT IS AMORTIZED TO INTEREST EXPENSE
  OVER THE TERM OF THE BOND, RESULTING IN
  HIGHER ANNUAL INTEREST EXPENSE THAN THE
  INTEREST PAID ON THE BOND.

- THE AMORTIZATION OF PREMIUM OR DISCOUNT
  RESULTS IN REPORTING AN ACTUAL INTEREST
  EXPENSE FROM THE BONDS THAT IS A FUNCTION
  OF THE MARKET INTEREST RATE WHEN THE BONDS
  WERE ISSUED -- AN APPROPRIATE RESULT.

DEFERRED INCOME TAXES

<u>WHAT'S GOING ON?</u>

· DIFFERENCES BETWEEN BOOK AND TAXABLE
  INCOME ARISE BECAUSE FINANCIAL ACCOUNTING
  METHODS DIFFER FROM ACCOUNTING METHODS
  PERMITTED FOR INCOME TAX PURPOSES.

  <u>EXAMPLE</u>: BOOK DEPRECIATION IS USUALLY
  CALCULATED ON A STRAIGHT-LINE BASIS, AND
  TAX DEPRECIATION IS USUALLY BASED ON AN
  ACCELERATED METHOD.

<u>KEY ISSUE</u>

· WHEN TAXABLE INCOME IS DIFFERENT FROM
  FINANCIAL ACCOUNTING (i.e., BOOK) INCOME,
  INCOME TAX EXPENSE SHOULD BE A FUNCTION
  OF BOOK INCOME BEFORE TAXES, NOT TAXABLE
  INCOME. THIS IS AN APPLICATION OF THE
  MATCHING CONCEPT.

<u>KEY IDEA</u>

· INCOME TAX EXPENSE BASED ON BOOK INCOME
  CAN BE MORE OR LESS THAN THE INCOME TAXES
  CURRENTLY PAYABLE. WHEN THIS OCCURS,

    · "DEFERRED INCOME TAX LIABILITIES" and/or

    · "DEFERRED INCOME TAX ASSETS"

  ARE REPORTED.

OWNERS' EQUITY - PAID-IN CAPITAL

ACCOUNTS INCLUDED IN PAID-IN CAPITAL

· COMMON STOCK (SOMETIMES CALLED CAPITAL STOCK)

· PREFERRED STOCK (IF AUTHORIZED BY THE CORPORATION'S CHARTER)

· ADDITIONAL PAID-IN CAPITAL

KEY TERMINOLOGY FOR NUMBER OF SHARES OF STOCK

· AUTHORIZED - BY THE CORPORATION'S CHARTER

· ISSUED - SOLD IN THE PAST TO STOCKHOLDERS

· OUTSTANDING - STILL HELD BY STOCKHOLDERS

· TREASURY STOCK - SHARES OF ITS OWN STOCK PURCHASED AND HELD BY THE CORPORATION. THE NUMBER OF SHARES OF TREASURY STOCK IS THE DIFFERENCE BETWEEN THE NUMBER OF SHARES ISSUED AND THE NUMBER OF SHARES OUTSTANDING.

KEY TERMINOLOGY FOR STOCK VALUE

· PAR VALUE - AN ARBITRARY AMOUNT ASSIGNED TO EACH SHARE AT INCORPORATION. THE FIRM CAN ISSUE NO-PAR VALUE STOCK. IF NO-PAR VALUE STOCK HAS A "STATED VALUE", THE STATED VALUE IS LIKE A PAR VALUE.

COMMON STOCK AND PREFERRED STOCK

KEY IDEAS

· COMMON STOCK REPRESENTS THE BASIC
  OWNERSHIP OF A CORPORATION.

· PREFERRED STOCK REPRESENTS OWNERSHIP, BUT
  HAS SOME PREFERENCES RELATIVE TO COMMON
  STOCK. THESE INCLUDE:

  · PRIORITY CLAIM TO DIVIDENDS, AND

  · PRIORITY CLAIM TO ASSETS IN LIQUIDATION.

  · HOWEVER, PREFERRED STOCKHOLDERS
    ARE NOT USUALLY ENTITLED TO VOTE FOR
    DIRECTORS.

KEY POINTS ABOUT DIVIDENDS ON PREFERRED STOCK

· DIVIDENDS ARE USUALLY "CUMULATIVE," WHICH
  MEANS THAT DIVIDENDS NOT PAID DURING ONE
  YEAR (IN ARREARS) MUST BE PAID IN A FUTURE
  YEAR BEFORE DIVIDENDS CAN BE PAID ON
  COMMON STOCK.

· DIVIDEND AMOUNT IS EXPRESSED AS A CERTAIN
  AMOUNT PER SHARE ($3.50), OR AS A PERCENT OF
  PAR VALUE (7% OF PAR VALUE OF $50).

PAID-IN CAPITAL AMOUNTS ON THE BALANCE SHEET

<u>WHAT'S GOING ON?</u>

- IF THE STOCK HAS A PAR VALUE, THE AMOUNTS OPPOSITE THE STOCK CAPTIONS ARE ALWAYS PAR VALUE MULTIPLIED BY THE NUMBER OF SHARES ISSUED.

- THE DIFFERENCE BETWEEN THE PAR VALUE AND THE AMOUNT RECEIVED PER SHARE WHEN THE STOCK WAS ISSUED IS RECORDED AS ADDITIONAL PAID-IN CAPITAL.

- IF THE STOCK IS NO-PAR VALUE STOCK (WITHOUT A STATED VALUE), THE AMOUNT OPPOSITE THE CAPTION IS THE TOTAL AMOUNT RECEIVED WHEN THE STOCK WAS ISSUED.

RETAINED EARNINGS AND DIVIDENDS

<u>KEY IDEAS</u>

· RETAINED EARNINGS INCREASES EACH PERIOD BY THE AMOUNT OF NET INCOME FOR THAT PERIOD. (NET LOSSES DECREASE RETAINED EARNINGS.)

· DIVIDENDS ARE DISTRIBUTIONS OF RETAINED EARNINGS TO THE STOCKHOLDERS, AND ARE A REDUCTION IN RETAINED EARNINGS.

> · CASH DIVIDENDS ARE DECLARED BY THE BOARD OF DIRECTORS AS AN AMOUNT PER SHARE.

> · STOCK DIVIDENDS ARE DECLARED BY THE BOARD OF DIRECTORS AS A PERCENTAGE OF THE PREVIOUSLY ISSUED SHARES. STOCK DIVIDENDS AFFECT ONLY RETAINED EARNINGS AND PAID-IN CAPITAL; ASSETS AND LIABILITIES ARE NOT AFFECTED.

> · CASH DIVIDENDS <u>ARE NOT</u> PAID ON TREASURY STOCK. STOCK DIVIDENDS <u>ARE</u> USUALLY ISSUED ON TREASURY STOCK.

STOCK SPLITS

KEY IDEA

- A STOCK SPLIT INVOLVES ISSUING ADDITIONAL SHARES OF STOCK IN PROPORTION TO THE NUMBER OF SHARES CURRENTLY OWNED BY EACH STOCKHOLDER. THE RELATIVE OWNERSHIP INTEREST OF EACH STOCKHOLDER DOES NOT CHANGE.

- BECAUSE THERE ARE MORE SHARES OF STOCK OUTSTANDING, THE MARKET PRICE OF EACH SHARE WILL FALL TO REFLECT THE SPLIT.

BALANCE SHEET EFFECT OF STOCK SPLIT

- DOLLAR AMOUNTS ON THE BALANCE SHEET ARE NOT AFFECTED. THE PAR VALUE IS REDUCED, AND THE NUMBER OF SHARES ISSUED IS INCREASED.

OTHER COMPREHENSIVE INCOME (LOSS)

HISTORICAL BACKGROUND

- ALTHOUGH OWNERS' EQUITY HAS CONSISTED OF TWO PRIMARY CATEGORIES (PAID-IN CAPITAL AND RETAINED EARNINGS), THERE HAS BEEN CONSIDERABLE DEBATE REGARDING WHICH ITEMS SHOULD BE ACCOUNTED FOR WITHIN "NET INCOME" VERSUS THOSE ITEMS THAT SHOULD BE ACCOUNTED FOR DIRECTLY WITHIN OWNERS' EQUITY.

KEY IDEA

- A NEW CATEGORY OF OWNERS' EQUITY—**OTHER COMPREHENSIVE INCOME (LOSS)**—WAS ESTABLISHED RECENTLY BY THE FASB TO HIGHLIGHT THE FOLLOWING _UNREALIZED_ CHANGES IN OWNERS' EQUITY:

  - CUMULATIVE FOREIGN CURRENCY TRANSLATION ADJUSTMENTS

  - UNREALIZED GAINS OR LOSSES ON AVAILABLE-FOR-SALE MARKETABLE SECURITIES

  - ADDITIONAL MINIMUM PENSION LIABILITY ADJUSTMENTS

KEY POINTS

- _**ALL**_ ITEMS OF INCOME (LOSS) ULTIMATELY AFFECT OWNERS' EQUITY ON THE BALANCE SHEET.

- THIS NEW CATEGORY OF OWNERS' EQUITY HAS IMPROVED COMPARABILITY BETWEEN FIRMS WHILE MAINTAINING FLEXIBILITY IN FINANCIAL REPORTING.

INCOME STATEMENT

MULTIPLE-STEP MODEL

CRUISERS, INC., AND SUBSIDIARIES
Consolidated Income Statement
For the Years Ended August 31, 2002, and 2001
(000 omitted)

	2002	2001
Net sales	$77,543	$62,531
Cost of goods sold	48,077	39,870
Gross profit	$29,466	$22,661
Selling, general, and administrative expenses	23,264	18,425
Income from operations	$ 6,202	$ 4,236
Other income (expense):		
Interest expense	(3,378)	(2,679)
Other income (net)	385	193
Minority interest	(432)	(356)
Income before taxes	$ 2,777	$ 1,394
Provision for income taxes	1,250	630
Net income	$ 1,527	$ 764
Basic earnings per share of common stock	$ 5.56	$ 2.42

KEY OBSERVATIONS

- THERE IS A GREAT DEAL OF SUMMARIZATION.

- CAPTIONS REFLECT THE REVENUE AND EXPENSE CATEGORIES THAT ARE MOST SIGNIFICANT TO UNDERSTANDING RESULTS OF OPERATIONS.

- INCOME FROM OPERATIONS IS SOMETIMES MORE MEANINGFUL FOR TREND COMPARISONS THAN NET INCOME.

LINKAGE BETWEEN BALANCE SHEET AND INCOME STATEMENT ACCOUNTS

BALANCE SHEET	INCOME STATEMENT
ACCOUNTS RECEIVABLE -------->	SALES / REVENUES
NOTES RECEIVABLE AND -------> SHORT-TERM INVESTMENTS	INTEREST INCOME
INVENTORIES ------------------------>	COST OF GOODS SOLD
PREPAID EXPENSES AND -------> ACCRUED LIABILITIES	OPERATING EXPENSES
ACCUMULATED ----------------------> DEPRECIATION	DEPRECIATION EXPENSE
	(REPORTED IN COST OF GOODS SOLD AND OPERATING EXPENSES)
NOTES PAYABLE AND ------------> BONDS PAYABLE	INTEREST EXPENSE
INCOME TAXES PAYABLE -------> AND DEFERRED TAX LIABILITY	INCOME TAX EXPENSE

STATEMENT OF CASH FLOWS

WHAT'S GOING ON?

· THE INCOME STATEMENT REPORTS ACCRUAL BASIS
  NET INCOME. FINANCIAL STATEMENT USERS ALSO
  WANT TO KNOW ABOUT THE FIRM'S CASH FLOWS.

· THE REASONS FOR THE CHANGE IN CASH FROM
  THE BEGINNING TO THE END OF THE PERIOD ARE
  SUMMARIZED IN THREE CATEGORIES:

  · CASH FLOWS FROM **OPERATING** ACTIVITIES

  · CASH FLOWS FROM **INVESTING** ACTIVITIES

  · CASH FLOWS FROM **FINANCING** ACTIVITIES

INTERPRETING THE STATEMENT OF CASH FLOWS

<u>KEY QUESTIONS</u>

- WHAT HAPPENED TO THE CASH BALANCE DURING
  THE YEAR?

- WHAT IS THE RELATIONSHIP BETWEEN CASH FLOWS
  FROM OPERATING, INVESTING, AND FINANCING
  ACTIVITIES?

<u>KEY RELATIONSHIPS TO OBSERVE</u>

- DID CASH FLOWS FROM OPERATING ACTIVITIES EXCEED
  CASH USED FOR INVESTING ACTIVITIES?

- DID FINANCING ACTIVITIES CAUSE A NET INCREASE OR
  NET DECREASE IN CASH?

- IN OPERATING ACTIVITIES, WHAT WERE THE EFFECTS OF
  ACCOUNTS RECEIVABLE, INVENTORY, AND ACCOUNTS
  PAYABLE CHANGES?

- IN INVESTING ACTIVITIES, WHAT WAS THE RELATIONSHIP
  BETWEEN THE INVESTMENT IN NEW ASSETS AND THE SALE
  OF OLD ASSETS?

- IN FINANCING ACTIVITIES, WHAT WERE THE NET EFFECTS
  OF LONG-TERM DEBT AND CAPITAL STOCK CHANGES?
  WHAT WAS THE EFFECT OF CASH DIVIDENDS PAID?

EXPLANATORY NOTES TO FINANCIAL STATEMENTS

KEY POINT

- FINANCIAL STATEMENT READERS MUST BE ABLE TO LEARN ABOUT THE FOLLOWING KEY ISSUES THAT AFFECT THEIR ABILITY TO UNDERSTAND THE STATEMENTS:

    - DEPRECIATION METHODS
    - INVENTORY COST FLOW ASSUMPTIONS
    - CURRENT AND DEFERRED INCOME TAXES
    - EMPLOYEE BENEFIT INFORMATION
    - EARNINGS PER SHARE OF COMMON STOCK DETAILS
    - STOCK OPTION AND STOCK PURCHASE PLAN INFORMATION

OTHER KEY DISCLOSURES

- MANAGEMENT'S STATEMENT OF RESPONSIBILITY
- MANAGEMENT'S DISCUSSION AND ANALYSIS

KEY IDEA

- THE EXPLANATORY NOTES TO THE FINANCIAL STATEMENTS MUST BE REVIEWED TO HAVE A REASONABLY COMPLETE UNDERSTANDING OF WHAT THE NUMBERS MEAN.

FIVE-YEAR (OR LONGER) SUMMARY OF FINANCIAL DATA

KEY IDEAS

- LOOK AT TREND OF DATA.

- NOTICE THE EFFECT OF STOCK DIVIDENDS AND STOCK SPLITS ON PER SHARE DATA.

- USE THE DATA REPORTED FOR PRIOR YEARS TO MAKE RATIO CALCULATIONS FOR EVALUATIVE PURPOSES.

INDEPENDENT AUDITORS' REPORT

KEY IDEA

- FINANCIAL STATEMENTS PRESENT FAIRLY, **IN ALL MATERIAL RESPECTS**, THE FINANCIAL POSITION AND RESULTS OF OPERATIONS.

KEY POINT

- AUDITORS GIVE NO GUARANTEE THAT FINANCIAL STATEMENTS ARE FREE FROM ERROR OR FRAUD.

LIQUIDITY ANALYSIS

KEY QUESTION

- IS THE FIRM LIKELY TO BE ABLE TO PAY ITS OBLIGATIONS WHEN THEY COME DUE?

LIQUIDITY MEASURES

- WORKING CAPITAL

- CURRENT RATIO

- ACID-TEST RATIO

KEY ISSUE

- THE INVENTORY COST FLOW ASSUMPTION USED BY THE FIRM (FIFO, LIFO, WEIGHTED AVERAGE, OR SPECIFIC IDENTIFICATION) WILL AFFECT THESE MEASURES.

ACTIVITY MEASURES

<u>KEY QUESTION</u>

· HOW EFFICIENTLY ARE THE FIRM'S ASSETS BEING USED?

<u>ACTIVITY MEASURES</u>

· ACCOUNTS RECEIVABLE TURNOVER (OR NUMBER OF DAYS' SALES IN ACCOUNTS RECEIVABLE)

· INVENTORY TURNOVER (OR NUMBER OF DAYS' SALES IN INVENTORY)

· PLANT AND EQUIPMENT TURNOVER

· TOTAL ASSET TURNOVER

<u>GENERAL MODEL</u>

$$\text{TURNOVER} = \frac{\text{SALES FOR PERIOD}}{\text{AVERAGE ASSET BALANCE FOR PERIOD}}$$

<u>KEY IDEAS</u>

· INVENTORY ACTIVITY CALCULATIONS USE COST OF GOODS SOLD INSTEAD OF SALES.

· NUMBER OF DAYS' SALES CALCULATIONS USE THE ENDING BALANCE OF THE ASSET ACCOUNT DIVIDED BY AVERAGE DAILY SALES OR AVERAGE DAILY COST OF GOODS SOLD.

PROFITABILITY MEASURES

<u>KEY QUESTIONS</u>

- WHAT RATE OF RETURN HAS BEEN EARNED ON ASSETS OR OWNERS' EQUITY?

- HOW EXPENSIVE IS THE FIRM'S COMMON STOCK RELATIVE TO OTHER COMPANIES, AND WHAT HAS BEEN THE DIVIDEND EXPERIENCE?

<u>PROFITABILITY MEASURES</u>

- ROI - RETURN ON INVESTMENT

- ROE - RETURN ON EQUITY

- PRICE / EARNINGS RATIO (EARNINGS MULTIPLE)

- DIVIDEND YIELD

- DIVIDEND PAYOUT RATIO

<u>KEY IDEAS</u>

- FACTORS IN ROI CALCULATION MAY DIFFER AMONG COMPANIES (NET INCOME OR OPERATING INCOME IN THE NUMERATOR); WHAT IS IMPORTANT IS THE CONSISTENCY OF DEFINITION, AND **TREND** OF ROI.

- ROE IS BASED ON THE NET INCOME APPLICABLE TO, AND THE EQUITY OF, **COMMON STOCKHOLDERS**.

FINANCIAL LEVERAGE RATIOS

<u>KEY IDEA</u>

· FINANCIAL LEVERAGE REFERS TO THE USE OF DEBT (INSTEAD OF OWNERS' EQUITY) TO FINANCE THE ACQUISITION OF ASSETS FOR THE FIRM.

THE INTEREST RATE ON DEBT IS FIXED, SO IF THE ROI EARNED ON THE BORROWED FUNDS IS GREATER THAN THE INTEREST RATE OWED, ROE WILL INCREASE. THIS IS REFERRED TO AS "POSITIVE" FINANCIAL LEVERAGE.

IF THE ROI EARNED ON BORROWED FUNDS IS LESS THAN THE INTEREST RATE OWED, ROE WILL DECREASE. THIS IS REFERRED TO AS "NEGATIVE" FINANCIAL LEVERAGE.

<u>KEY QUESTIONS</u>

· HOW MUCH FINANCIAL LEVERAGE IS THE FIRM USING?

· HOW MUCH RISK OF FINANCIAL LOSS TO CREDITORS AND OWNERS IS THERE?

<u>FINANCIAL LEVERAGE RATIOS</u>

· DEBT RATIO

· DEBT / EQUITY RATIO

· TIMES INTEREST EARNED RATIO

63

OTHER ANALYTICAL TECHNIQUES

BOOK VALUE PER SHARE OF COMMON STOCK

KEY IDEA

· AN EASILY CALCULATED AMOUNT BASED ON THE BALANCE SHEET AMOUNT OF OWNERS' EQUITY, BUT NOT VERY USEFUL IN MOST CASES BECAUSE BALANCE SHEET AMOUNTS DO NOT REFLECT MARKET VALUES OR REPLACEMENT VALUES.

COMMON SIZE FINANCIAL STATEMENTS

KEY IDEA

· COMPARISONS BETWEEN FIRMS (OR BETWEEN PERIODS FOR THE SAME FIRM) CAN BE MORE EASILY UNDERSTOOD IF FINANCIAL STATEMENT AMOUNTS ARE EXPRESSED AS PERCENTAGES OF TOTAL ASSETS OR TOTAL REVENUES.

OTHER OPERATING STATISTICS

KEY IDEA

· NOT ALL DECISIONS AND INFORMED JUDGMENTS ABOUT AN ENTITY ARE BASED ON FINANCIAL DATA. NONFINANCIAL STATISTICS ARE FREQUENTLY RELEVANT AND USEFUL.

MANAGERIAL ACCOUNTING COMPARED TO FINANCIAL ACCOUNTING

KEY CHARACTERISTICS THAT DIFFER

- SERVICE PERSPECTIVE

- BREADTH OF CONCERN

- REPORTING FREQUENCY AND PROMPTNESS

- DEGREE OF PRECISION OF DATA USED

- REPORTING STANDARDS

COST CLASSIFICATIONS

KEY IDEA
· DIFFERENT COSTS FOR DIFFERENT PURPOSES.

COST CLASSIFICATIONS

· FOR COST ACCOUNTING PURPOSES (CH 12, 14, & 15):
    · PRODUCT COST
    · PERIOD COST

· RELATIONSHIP TO PRODUCT OR ACTIVITY (CH 13):
    · DIRECT COST
    · INDIRECT COST

· RELATIONSHIP BETWEEN TOTAL COST AND
VOLUME OF ACTIVITY (CH 13):
    · VARIABLE COST
    · FIXED COST

· TIME-FRAME PERSPECTIVE (CH 14 & 15):
    · COMMITTED COST
    · DISCRETIONARY COST
    · CONTROLLABLE COST
    · NONCONTROLLABLE COST

· FOR OTHER ANALYTICAL PURPOSES (CH 16):
    · DIFFERENTIAL COST
    · ALLOCATED COST
    · SUNK COST
    · OPPORTUNITY COST

RELATIONSHIP OF TOTAL COST TO VOLUME OF ACTIVITY

KEY IDEA

- **COST BEHAVIOR PATTERN** DESCRIBES HOW TOTAL COST VARIES WITH CHANGES IN ACTIVITY.

KEY RELATIONSHIPS

- VARIABLE COST
- FIXED COST

EXHIBIT 12–3 Cost Behavior Patterns

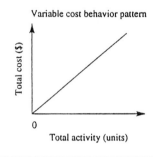

Variable cost behavior pattern

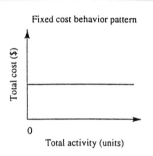

Fixed cost behavior pattern

KEY ASSUMPTIONS

- RELEVANT RANGE

- LINEARITY

COST FORMULA

<u>KEY POINT</u>

- A **COST FORMULA** DESCRIBES THE EXPECTED TOTAL COST FOR ANY VOLUME OF ACTIVITY, USING COST BEHAVIOR INFORMATION.

<u>KEY RELATIONSHIP</u>

- TOTAL COST = FIXED COST + VARIABLE COST

    = FIXED COST + (VARIABLE RATE
                         PER UNIT * ACTIVITY)

<u>KEY IDEA</u>

- WHENEVER POSSIBLE, AVOID UNITIZING FIXED COSTS, BECAUSE THEY DO NOT BEHAVE THAT WAY!

INCOME STATEMENT MODELS

TRADITIONAL MODEL

```
  REVENUES
- COST OF GOODS SOLD
  GROSS PROFIT
- OPERATING EXPENSES
  OPERATING INCOME
```

CONTRIBUTION MARGIN MODEL

```
  REVENUES
- VARIABLE EXPENSES
  CONTRIBUTION MARGIN
- FIXED EXPENSES
  OPERATING INCOME
```

KEY IDEAS

· THE TRADITIONAL MODEL CLASSIFIES EXPENSES
  BY FUNCTION, AND THE CONTRIBUTION MARGIN
  MODEL CLASSIFIES EXPENSES BY COST
  BEHAVIOR PATTERN.

· THE CONTRIBUTION MARGIN MODEL IS USEFUL
  FOR DETERMINING THE EFFECT ON OPERATING
  INCOME OF CHANGES IN THE LEVEL OF ACTIVITY.

EXPANDED CONTRIBUTION MARGIN MODEL

	PER UNIT	X	VOLUME	=	TOTAL	%
REVENUE	$ **1.**				$	100%
VARIABLE EXP.	**1.**					
CONT. MARGIN	$ **1.**	X	**2.**	=	**2.**	
FIXED EXPENSES					**3.**	
OPERATING INCOME					$ **3.**	

KEY IDEAS

· THE PREFERRED ROUTE THROUGH THE MODEL IS:

1. TO ENTER PER UNIT REVENUE AND VARIABLE
   EXPENSES TO GET UNIT CONTRIBUTION MARGIN.

2. THEN MULTIPLY UNIT CONTRIBUTION MARGIN
   BY VOLUME (QUANTITY SOLD) TO GET TOTAL
   CONTRIBUTION MARGIN.

3. FIXED EXPENSES ARE NOT EXPRESSED ON A PER
   UNIT BASIS; THEY ARE SUBTRACTED FROM TOTAL
   CONTRIBUTION MARGIN TO GET OPERATING
   INCOME.

· THE CONTRIBUTION MARGIN RATIO EXPRESSES
  CONTRIBUTION MARGIN AS A PERCENTAGE OF
  REVENUES, ON EITHER A PER UNIT OR TOTAL BASIS.

BREAK-EVEN POINT ANALYSIS

KEY IDEA

· MANAGERS FREQUENTLY WANT TO KNOW THE
  NUMBER OF UNITS THAT MUST BE SOLD, OR THE
  TOTAL SALES DOLLARS REQUIRED, TO BREAK-EVEN
  (HAVE ZERO OPERATING INCOME).

BREAK-EVEN GRAPH

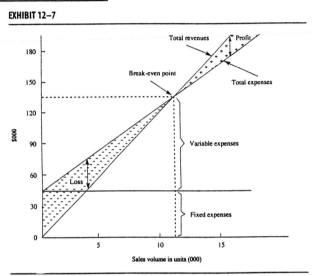

EXHIBIT 12–7

KEY POINT

· ONCE THE BREAK-EVEN POINT HAS BEEN REACHED,
  OPERATING INCOME INCREASES BY THE AMOUNT
  OF CONTRIBUTION MARGIN FROM EACH ADDITIONAL
  UNIT SOLD.

KEY ASSUMPTIONS TO REMEMBER WHEN USING CONTRIBUTION MARGIN ANALYSIS

· COST BEHAVIOR PATTERNS CAN BE IDENTIFIED.

· COSTS ARE LINEAR WITHIN THE RELEVANT RANGE.

· ACTIVITY REMAINS WITHIN THE RELEVANT RANGE.

· SALES MIX OF THE FIRM'S PRODUCTS WITH DIFFERENT CONTRIBUTION MARGIN RATIOS DOES NOT CHANGE.

KEY POINT

· IF THESE SIMPLIFYING ASSUMPTIONS ARE NOT VALID, THE ANALYSIS IS MADE MORE COMPLICATED BUT THE CONCEPTS ARE STILL APPLICABLE.

COST MANAGEMENT

KEY IDEAS

- COST INFORMATION FROM THE ACCOUNTING SYSTEM IS USED TO MANAGE THE ACTIVITIES OF THE ORGANIZATION.

- VALUE CHAIN FUNCTIONS

  - RESEARCH AND DEVELOPMENT
  - DESIGN
  - PRODUCTION
  - MARKETING
  - DISTRIBUTION
  - CUSTOMER SERVICE

COST ACCUMULATION AND ASSIGNMENT

KEY CONCEPTS

- COST OBJECT

- COST ACCUMULATION → COST POOL

- COST ASSIGNMENT → COST OBJECT

COST ACCOUNTING SYSTEMS

KEY IDEAS

· PERIOD COSTS (SELLING, GENERAL, AND ADMIN-
ISTRATIVE) ARE ACCOUNTED FOR AS EXPENSES IN
THE PERIOD INCURRED.

· PRODUCT COSTS FLOW THROUGH INVENTORY (ASSET)
ACCOUNTS, AND THEN TO THE COST OF GOODS SOLD
(EXPENSE) ACCOUNT.

RAW MATERIAL, DIRECT LABOR, AND **MANUFACTURING
OVERHEAD** COSTS ARE CAPITALIZED AS INVENTORY →
UNTIL THE PRODUCT THEY RELATE TO IS SOLD.

   · RAW MATERIAL AND DIRECT LABOR COSTS ARE
   RATHER EASILY IDENTIFIED WITH THE PRODUCT.

   · MANUFACTURING OVERHEAD IS "APPLIED" TO
   PRODUCTION BASED ON A **PREDETERMINED
   OVERHEAD APPLICATION RATE**, DETERMINED
   AS FOLLOWS:

> ESTIMATED OVERHEAD COSTS FOR THE YEAR
> ESTIMATED ACTIVITY FOR THE YEAR

KEY POINT

BECAUSE THE PREDETERMINED OVERHEAD APPLI-CATION
RATE IS BASED ON ESTIMATES, THERE WILL PROBABLY BE
"OVERAPPLIED" OR "UNDERAPPLIED" OVERHEAD AT THE
END OF THE YEAR. THIS AMOUNT USUALLY BECOMES
PART OF COST OF GOODS SOLD.

COST OF GOODS MANUFACTURED AND COST OF GOODS SOLD

<u>KEY IDEA</u>

· BECAUSE OF THE INVENTORY ACCOUNTS, COST OF GOODS MANUFACTURED AND COST OF GOODS SOLD ARE NOT SIMPLY THE TOTALS OF COSTS INCURRED DURING THE PERIOD.

<u>KEY MODELS</u>

· COST OF GOODS MANUFACTURED:

    RAW MATERIALS INVENTORY, BEGINNING
+ RAW MATERIALS PURCHASES
- <u>RAW MATERIALS INVENTORY, ENDING</u>
= COST OF RAW MATERIALS USED
+ WORK-IN-PROCESS INVENTORY, BEGINNING
+ DIRECT LABOR COSTS INCURRED
+ MANUFACTURING OVERHEAD APPLIED
- <u>WORK-IN-PROCESS INVENTORY, ENDING</u>
= COST OF GOODS MANUFACTURED

· COST OF GOODS SOLD:

    FINISHED GOODS INVENTORY, BEGINNING
+ COST OF GOODS MANUFACTURED
- <u>FINISHED GOODS INVENTORY, ENDING</u>
= COST OF GOODS SOLD

ACTIVITY BASED COSTING

<u>KEY POINT</u>

- AN ABC SYSTEM INVOLVES IDENTIFYING THE KEY
  ACTIVITIES THAT CAUSE THE INCURRANCE OF COST;
  THESE ACTIVITIES ARE KNOWN AS **COST DRIVERS.**

- EXAMPLES OF COST DRIVERS INCLUDE: MACHINE
  SETUP, QUALITY INSPECTION, PRODUCTION ORDER
  PREPARATION, AND MATERIALS HANDLING ACTIVITIES.

<u>KEY RELATIONSHIPS</u>

- THE NUMBER OF TIMES EACH ACTIVITY IS TO BE
  PERFORMED DURING THE YEAR AND THE TOTAL
  COST OF EACH ACTIVITY ARE ESTIMATED, AND A
  PREDETERMINED COST PER ACTIVITY IS
  CALCULATED.

- "ACTIVITY BASED COSTS" ARE THEN APPLIED TO
  PRODUCTS, RATHER THAN USING A TRADITIONAL
  METHOD OF OVERHEAD APPLICATION SUCH AS
  DIRECT LABOR HOURS OR MACHINE HOURS.

<u>KEY IDEA</u>

- ABC SYSTEMS OFTEN LEAD TO MORE ACCURATE
  PRODUCT COSTING AND MORE EFFECTIVE COST
  CONTROL, BECAUSE MANAGEMENT'S ATTENTION
  IS DIRECTED TO THE ACTIVITIES THAT *CAUSE*
  THE INCURRANCE OF COST.

BUDGETING

BUDGET CATEGORIES

- OPERATING BUDGET

- CAPITAL BUDGET

APPROACHES TO BUDGETING

- TOP-DOWN

- PARTICIPATIVE

- ZERO-BASED

BUDGET TIME FRAMES

- SINGLE-PERIOD BUDGET

- ROLLING (CONTINUOUS) BUDGET

OPERATING BUDGET PREPARATION SEQUENCE

- SALES / REVENUE BUDGET, OR SALES FORECAST

- PURCHASES / PRODUCTION BUDGET

- OPERATING EXPENSE BUDGET

- BUDGETED INCOME STATEMENT

- CASH BUDGET

- BALANCE SHEET BUDGET

KEY POINT

- THE ENTIRE BUDGET BUILDS ON THE SALES/ REVENUE BUDGET, SOMETIMES CALLED THE SALES FORECAST.

STANDARD COSTS

<u>WHAT ARE THEY?</u>

- UNIT BUDGETS FOR MATERIALS, LABOR, AND OVERHEAD COST COMPONENTS OF A PRODUCT OR PROCESS.

- STANDARD COSTS ARE USED FOR PLANNING AND CONTROL.

<u>KEY IDEAS</u>

- STANDARD COSTS CAN BE BASED ON:

    - IDEAL, OR ENGINEERED, PERFORMANCE

    - ATTAINABLE PERFORMANCE

    - PAST EXPERIENCE

- THE STANDARD COST OF PRODUCT OR PROCESS COMPONENTS CAN BE USED TO BUILD UP THE TOTAL COST OF A PRODUCT OR PROCESS.

PERFORMANCE REPORTING

KEY IDEAS

- IF TIME AND EFFORT HAVE BEEN EXPENDED PREPARING A BUDGET, IT IS APPROPRIATE TO COMPARE ACTUAL RESULTS WITH BUDGETED RESULTS. THIS IS DONE IN THE PERFORMANCE REPORT.

- IF ACTUAL RESULTS APPROXIMATE BUDGETED RESULTS, THEN NO SIGNIFICANT FURTHER EVALUATION OF PERFORMANCE NEEDS TO BE MADE.

- MANAGEMENT ATTENTION IS GIVEN ONLY TO THOSE ACTIVITIES FOR WHICH ACTUAL RESULTS VARY SIGNIFICANTLY FROM BUDGETED RESULTS. THIS IS **MANAGEMENT BY EXCEPTION.**

SEGMENT REPORTING

<u>KEY IDEAS</u>

- · WHEN A FIRM HAS SEVERAL IDENTIFIABLE SEGMENTS (DIVISIONS, SALES TERRITORIES, PRODUCTS, ETC.) MANAGEMENT FREQUENTLY WANTS TO EVALUATE THE OPERATING RESULTS OF EACH SEGMENT.

- · SEGMENTS MAY BE REFERRED TO AS:

    - · COST CENTERS

    - · PROFIT CENTERS

    - · INVESTMENT CENTERS

<u>KEY ISSUES</u>

- · SALES, VARIABLE EXPENSES, AND CONTRIBUTION MARGIN FOR EACH SEGMENT CAN USUALLY BE EASILY ACCUMULATED FROM THE ACCOUNTING RECORDS.

- · FIXED EXPENSES INCLUDE AMOUNTS ASSOCIATED DIRECTLY WITH EACH SEGMENT, AND AMOUNTS THAT ARE COMMON TO THE FIRM AS A WHOLE.

- · TO REPORT SENSIBLE RESULTS FOR EACH SEGMENT, **COMMON FIXED EXPENSES SHOULD NEVER BE ARBITRARILY ALLOCATED TO THE SEGMENTS** BECAUSE THEY ARE NOT INCURRED DIRECTLY BY ANY OF THE SEGMENTS.

FLEXIBLE BUDGETING

KEY ISSUES

· BUDGET AMOUNTS ARE BASED ON EXPECTED LEVELS
  OF ACTIVITY. ACTUAL ACTIVITY IS UNLIKELY TO BE THE
  SAME AS BUDGETED ACTIVITY.

· SOME MANAGER IS RESPONSIBLE FOR THE DIFFERENCE
  BETWEEN BUDGETED AND ACTUAL ACTIVITY LEVELS,
  BUT IT IS USUALLY ANOTHER MANAGER WHO IS
  RESPONSIBLE FOR THE COSTS INCURRED.

· REVENUES ARE A FUNCTION OF UNITS SOLD, AND
  COSTS INCURRED ARE A FUNCTION OF COST
  BEHAVIOR PATTERNS.

KEY IDEA

· AT THE END OF A PERIOD, WHEN THE ACTUAL LEVEL
  OF ACTIVITY IS KNOWN, THE ORIGINAL BUDGET SHOULD
  BE **FLEXED** SO THAT THE PERFORMANCE REPORT
  COMPARES ACTUAL RESULTS WITH BUDGET AMOUNTS
  BASED ON ACTUAL ACTIVITY.

KEY POINT

· ONLY REVENUES AND VARIABLE EXPENSES ARE
  FLEXED. FIXED EXPENSES ARE NOT A FUNCTION OF
  THE LEVEL OF ACTIVITY (UNLESS ACTIVITY FALLS
  OUTSIDE OF THE RELEVANT RANGE).

VARIABLE COST VARIANCE ANALYSIS

KEY IDEAS

· IT IS APPROPRIATE TO EVALUATE PERFORMANCE BY
  COMPARING ACTUAL COSTS WITH STANDARD COSTS,
  AND ANALYZING WHY ANY VARIANCES OCCURRED.

· THE REASON FOR CALCULATING VARIANCES IS TO
  ENCOURAGE ACTION TO ELIMINATE UNFAVORABLE
  VARIANCES AND CAPTURE FAVORABLE VARIANCES.

KEY POINTS

· VARIANCE TERMINOLOGY:

INPUT	QUANTITY VARIANCE	COST PER UNIT OF INPUT VARIANCE
RAW MATERIALS	USAGE	PRICE
DIRECT LABOR	EFFICIENCY	RATE
VAR. OVERHEAD	EFFICIENCY	SPENDING

· DIFFERENT MANAGERS ARE USUALLY RESPONSIBLE
  FOR THE QUANTITY AND COST PER UNIT OF INPUT
  VARIANCES. THAT IS WHY THEY ARE CALCULATED
  AND REPORTED SEPARATELY.

· THE REPORTING OF VARIANCES SHOULD LEAD TO
  BETTER COMMUNICATION AND COORDINATION OF
  ACTIVITIES.

FIXED COST VARIANCE ANALYSIS

<u>KEY ISSUE</u>

· FOR MANY FIRMS, FIXED MANUFACTURING OVERHEAD HAS BECOME MORE SIGNIFICANT THAN VARIABLE MANUFACTURING COSTS. THEREFORE, MANY FIRMS ARE INCREASING EFFORTS TO CONTROL FIXED OVERHEAD.

<u>KEY POINTS</u>

· VARIANCE TERMINOLOGY:

  · **BUDGET VARIANCE** IS THE DIFFERENCE BETWEEN BUDGETED FIXED OVERHEAD COSTS AND ACTUAL FIXED OVERHEAD COSTS.

  · **VOLUME VARIANCE** IS CAUSED BY THE DIFFERENCE BETWEEN THE PLANNED LEVEL OF ACTIVITY USED IN THE CALCULATION OF THE PREDETERMINED OVERHEAD APPLICATION RATE, AND THE ACTUAL LEVEL OF ACTIVITY.

  · THE SUM OF THE BUDGET VARIANCE AND THE VOLUME VARIANCE EQUALS THE OVERAPPLIED OR UNDERAPPLIED FIXED MANUFACTURING OVERHEAD.

DECISION MAKING

WHAT'S GOING ON?

- ENCOMPASES THE ENTIRE PLANNING AND CONTROL CYCLE

KEY COST CONCEPTS

- DIFFERENTIAL COST
- ALLOCATED COST
- SUNK COST
- OPPORTUNITY COST

SHORT-RUN DECISION ANALYSIS

KEY ISSUE

- ONLY THOSE FUTURE COSTS THAT REPRESENT DIFFERENCES BETWEEN DECISION ALTERNATIVES ARE CONSIDERED TO BE **RELEVANT COSTS**

SPECIAL PRICING DECISIONS

KEY QUESTION

- IS THE FIRM OPERATING AT FULL OR IDLE CAPACITY?

CAPITAL BUDGETING

WHAT'S GOING ON?

· PROPOSED CAPITAL EXPENDITURES USUALLY INVOLVE RETURNS RECEIVED OVER EXTENDED PERIODS OF TIME, SO IT IS APPROPRIATE TO RECOGNIZE THE TIME VALUE OF MONEY WHEN EVALUATING WHETHER OR NOT THE INVESTMENT WILL GENERATE THE DESIRED ROI.

KEY POINT

· PRESENT VALUE ANALYSIS RECOGNIZES THE TIME VALUE OF MONEY.

KEY ISSUE

· PRESENT VALUE ANALYSIS USES:

   1. THE INVESTMENT AMOUNT
   2. THE EXPECTED CASH RETURNS, AND
   3. AN INTEREST RATE (COST OF CAPITAL),

   TO ANSWER THE FOLLOWING QUESTION:

> IS THE PRESENT VALUE OF THE FUTURE CASH FLOWS FROM THE INVESTMENT, DISCOUNTED AT THE COST OF CAPITAL, AT LEAST EQUAL TO THE AMOUNT THAT MUST BE INVESTED?

   IF THE ANSWER IS "YES", THEN THE ROI ON THE CAPITAL EXPENDITURE IS AT LEAST EQUAL TO THE COST OF CAPITAL, AND THE INVESTMENT SHOULD BE MADE.

86

CAPITAL BUDGETING ANALYSIS TECHNIQUES

METHODS THAT USE PRESENT VALUE ANALYSIS

· NET PRESENT VALUE (NPV) METHOD:

  · GIVEN A COST OF CAPITAL, COMPUTE THE PRESENT
    VALUE OF THE CASH RETURNS FROM THE INVESTMENT
    AND THEN SUBTRACT THE INVESTMENT REQUIRED.
    THIS DIFFERENCE IS THE NET PRESENT VALUE (NPV)
    OF THE PROJECT:

  > · IF THE NPV IS POSITIVE, ROI > COST OF CAPITAL,
  >   SO THE INVESTMENT SHOULD BE MADE.
  >
  > · IF THE NPV IS NEGATIVE, ROI < COST OF CAPITAL,
  >   SO THE INVESTMENT SHOULD NOT BE MADE.
  >
  > · IF THE NPV IS ZERO, ROI = COST OF CAPITAL,
  >   SO THE FIRM WOULD BE INDIFFERENT ABOUT
  >   THE INVESTMENT PROPOSAL.

· INTERNAL RATE OF RETURN (IRR) METHOD:

  · SOLVE FOR THE INTEREST RATE AT WHICH THE
    PRESENT VALUE OF THE CASH RETURNS EQUALS
    THE INVESTMENT REQUIRED. THIS IS THE PROPOSED
    INVESTMENT'S ROI -- REFERRED TO AS THE INTERNAL
    RATE OF RETURN (IRR).

  · THE INVESTMENT DECISION IS MADE BASED ON THE
    RELATIONSHIP BETWEEN THE PROJECT'S INTERNAL
    RATE OF RETURN (IRR) AND THE FIRM'S DESIRED ROI
    (COST OF CAPITAL).

87

CAPITAL BUDGETING ANALYSIS TECHNIQUES

METHODS THAT DO NOT USE PRESENT VALUE ANALYSIS

· PAYBACK METHOD:

> HOW LONG DOES IT TAKE FOR THE CASH FLOWS
> TO EQUAL THE AMOUNT OF THE INVESTMENT?

· ACCOUNTING RATE OF RETURN METHOD:

> WHAT IS THE ROI BASED ON FINANCIAL STATEMENT
> REPORTING OF THE INVESTMENT AND OPERATING
> RESULTS?

KEY ISSUE

· THESE METHODS ARE SIGNIFICANTLY FLAWED BECAUSE
THEY IGNORE THE TIME VALUE OF MONEY.

Accounting—Present and Past

E1-5. The principal factors Marsha Thompson must consider are her competence and independence. Is she competent to prepare financial statements for a company that operates in a different industry than the one in which she works? A contingent fee arrangement would normally be considered an impairment of her independence because she would directly benefit if the loan were to be approved.

E1-7. Answers will vary depending on the browsers used by students to locate the requested information.

CHAPTER 2

Financial Statements and Accounting Concepts/Principles

E2-1.

	Category	Financial Statement(s)
Cash	A	BS
Accounts payable.......	L	BS
Common stock	OE	BS
Depreciation expense.	E	IS
Net sales.......	R	IS
Income tax expense	E	IS
Short-term investments.............................	A	BS
Gain on sale of land	G	IS
Retained earnings.......	OE	BS
Dividends payable.......	L	BS
Accounts receivable...	A	BS
Short-term debt	L	BS

E2-3. Use the accounting equation to solve for the missing information.

Firm A:

```
    A    =    L    +   PIC   + ( Beg. RE  + NI -  DIV     = End. RE )
$420,000 = $215,000 + $75,000 + ( $78,000  +  ? - $50,000 =    ?     )
```

In this case, the ending balance of retained earnings must be determined first:
$420,000 = $215,000 + $75,000 + End. RE.
Retained earnings, 12/31/02 = **$130,000**

Once the ending balance of retained earnings is known, net income can be determined:
$78,000 + NI - $50,000 = $130,000
Net income for 2002 = **$102,000**

Firm B:

```
    A    =    L    +  PIC  + (  Beg.RE +  NI        -   DIV    = End. RE )
$540,000 = $145,000 +   ?   + (    ?    + $83,000 - $19,000 = $310,000 )
```

$540,000 = $145,000 + PIC + $310,000
Paid-in capital, 12/31/02 = **$85,000**

Beg. RE + $83,000 – $19,000 = $310,000
Retained earnings, 1/1/02 = **$246,000**

E2-3. *(continued)*

Firm C:

```
   A    =  L  +    PIC   + (  Beg.RE  +    NI     -    DIV   = End. RE )
$325,000 =  ?  + $40,000 + ( $42,000 + $113,000 - $65,000 =    ?       )
```

In this case, the ending balance of retained earnings must be determined first:
$42,000 + $113,000 - $65,000 = End. RE
Retained earnings, 12/31/02 = **$90,000**

Once the ending balance of retained earnings is known, liabilities can be determined:
$325,000 = L + $40,000 + $90,000
Total liabilities, 12/31/02 = **$195,000**

E2-5. Prepare the retained earnings portion of a statement of changes in owners' equity for the year ended December 31, 2002:

Retained earnings, December 31, 2001	$311,800
Less: Net loss for the year ended December 31, 2002	(4,700)
Less: Dividends declared and paid in 2001....	(18,500)
Retained earnings, December 31, 2001	**$288,600**

E2-7.

```
                                         |        OE
               A    =    L    +   PIC    +     RE
Beginning: $12,400 = $7,000  + $  0  +   $5,400
Changes:       ?   = -1,200  +    0  +    3,000 (net income)
                                              (dividends)
Ending:        ?   =    ?    +     0  +   $6,000
```

Solution approach:
*(Remember that **net assets** = Assets – Liabilities = Owners' equity = PIC + RE).*
Since paid-in capital did not change during the year, assume that the beginning and ending balances are $0. Thus, beginning retained earnings = $12,400 – $7,000 = **$5,400**, and ending retained earnings = net assets at the end of the year = **$6,000**. By looking at the RE column, it can be seen that dividends must have been **$2,400**. Also by looking at the liabilities column, it can be seen that ending liabilities are **$5,800**, and therefore ending assets must be **$11,800**. Thus, total assets decreased by **$600** during the year ($12,400 – $11,800), which is equal to the net decrease on the right-hand side of the balance sheet (–$1,200 liabilities + $3,000 net income –$2,400 dividends = $600 net decrease in assets).

P2-9. Set up the accounting equation and show the effects of the transactions described. Since total assets must equal total liabilities and owners' equity, the *unadjusted* owners' equity can be calculated by subtracting liabilities from the total of the assets given.

	Cash	+ Inventory	+ Accounts Receivable	+ Plant & Equipment =	Liabilities	+ Owners' Equity
			A		**L** +	**OE**
Data given	$22,800 +	61,400	+ 114,200	+ 265,000 =	305,600	+ 157,800
Liquidation of inventory *	+49,120	−61,400				−12,280
Collection of acc. rec. *	+108,490		−114,200			−5,710
Sale of plant & equipment *	+190,000			−265,000		−75,000
Payment of liabilities	−305,600				−305,600	
Balance	$ 64,810 +	0	+ 0	+ 0 =	0	+ $ 64,810

* The effects of these transactions on owners' equity represent losses from the sale (or collection) of the non-cash assets.

P2-11. a. Accounts receivable .... $ 33,000
   Cash 9,000
   Supplies 6,000
   Merchandise inventory 31,000
   Total current assets .... **$ 79,000**

b. Accounts payable .... $ 23,000
   Long-term debt 40,000
   Common stock..... 10,000
   Retained earnings. 59,000
   Total liabilities and owners' equity **$132,000**

c. Sales revenue........ .... $140,000
   Cost of goods sold .... (90,000)
   Gross profit......... .... $ 50,000
   Service revenue 20,000
   Depreciation expense .... (12,000)
   Supplies expense .. .. (14,000)
   Earnings from operations (operating income) .... **$ 44,000**

P2-11. d.

Earnings from operations (operating income)	$ 44,000
Interest expense	(4,000)
Earnings before taxes	$ 40,000
Income tax expense	(12,000)
Net income	**$ 28,000**

e. $12,000 income tax expense / $40,000 earnings before taxes = **30% tax rate**

f.

Retained earnings, January 1, 2002	?
Net income for the year	$ 28,000
Dividends declared and paid during the year	(16,000)
Retained earnings, December 31, 2002	$ 59,000

Solving the model, the beginning retained earnings balance must have been **$47,000**, because the account balance increased by $12,000 during the year to an ending balance of $59,000.

P2-13. a.

BREANNA, INC.
Income Statement
For the Year Ended December 31, 2002

Sales	$200,000
Cost of goods sold	(128,000)
Gross profit	$ 72,000
Selling, general, and administrative expenses	(34,000)
Earnings from operations (operating income)	$ 38,000
Interest expense	(6,000)
Earnings before taxes	$ 32,000
Income tax expense	(8,000)
Net income	$ 24,000

BREANNA, INC.
Statement of Changes in Owners' Equity
For the Year Ended December 31, 2002

Paid-in capital:		
Common stock		$ 90,000
Retained earnings:		
Beginning balance	$ 23,000	
Net income for the year	24,000	
Less: Dividends declared and paid during the year	(12,000)	
Ending balance		35,000
Total owners' equity		$125,000

P2-13. a. *(continued)*

BREANNA, INC.
Balance Sheet
December 31, 2002

Assets:

Cash	$ 65,000	
Accounts receivable	10,000	
Merchandise inventory	37,000	
Total current assets		$112,000
Equipment.........	120,000	
Less: Accumulated depreciation	(52,000)	68,000
Total assets		$180,000

Liabilities:

Accounts payable	$ 15,000	
Long-term debt	40,000	
Total liabilities...		$ 55,000

Owners' Equity:

Common stock	$ 90,000	
Retained earnings	35,000	
Total owners' equity		$125,000
Total liabilities and owners' equity........		$180,000

b. $8,000 income tax expense / $32,000 earnings before taxes = **25% tax rate.**

c. $6,000 interest expense / $40,000 long-term debt = **15% interest rate.** This assumes that the year-end balance of long-term debt is representative of the *average* long-term debt account balance throughout the year.

d. $90,000 common stock / 9,000 shares = **$10 per share par value.**

e. $12,000 dividends declared and paid/ $24,000 net income = **50%.** This assumes that the board of directors has a policy to pay dividends in proportion to earnings.

P2-15. a.

Retained earnings, January 1, 2002...........	$ 75,000
Net income for the year...............	?
Dividends declared and paid during the year........	(17,000)
Retained earnings, December 31, 2002.....	$ 70,000

Solving for the missing amount, net income for the year is **$12,000.**

Revenues...	$120,000
Expenses...	?
Net income	$ 12,000

Solving for the missing amount, total expenses for the year are **$108,000.**

P2-15. b.

GARBER, INC.
Statement of Cash Flows
For the Year Ended December 31, 2002

Cash flows from operating activities................	$ 27,000
Cash flows from investing activities................	0
Cash flows from financing activities	(12,000)
Net increase in cash for the year..	$ 15,000
Cash balance, January 1, 2002......	35,000
Cash balance, December 31, 2002	$ 50,000

c. Depreciation expense of $15,000 was added back to net income to arrive at the cash flows from operating activities. (Since no production equipment was purchased or sold during the year, the $15,000 decrease in net production equipment is attributable to depreciation expense.)

d. Issuance of common stock...........	$ 10,000
Repayment of long-term debt	(5,000)
Payment of cash dividends...........	(17,000)
Net cash used for financing activities	$(12,000)

e. Garber, Inc., is better off at the end of the year. Although total assets did not change during the year, liabilities decreased by $5,000 and total owners' equity increased by $5,000. Net income of $12,000 was earned, and this is the bottom-line measure of profitability. In addition, the firm generated $27,000 in cash flows from operations and $10,000 from the sale of common stock (a financing activity). These cash flows allowed Garber, Inc., to reduce its long-term debt by $5,000, pay dividends of $17,000, and still have a net increase in cash of $15,000.

P2-17.

		Assets	*= Liabilities*	*Owners'* *+ Equity*
a.	Borrowed cash on a bank loan	+	+	NE
b.	Paid an account payable	-	-	NE
c.	Sold common stock	+	NE	+
d.	Purchased merchandise inventory on account	+	+	NE
e.	Declared and paid dividends	-	NE	-
f.	Collected an account receivable	NE	NE	NE
g.	Sold inventory on account at a profit	+	NE	+
h.	Paid operating expenses in cash	-	NE	-
i.	Repaid principal and interest on a bank loan	-	-	-

P2-19. Amounts shown in the balance sheet below reflect the following use of the data given:

a. An asset should have a "probable future economic benefit"; therefore the accounts receivable are stated at the amount expected to be collected from customers.
b. Assets are reported at original cost, not current "worth." Depreciation in accounting reflects the spreading of the cost of an asset over its estimated useful life.
c. Assets are reported at original cost, not at an assessed or appraised value.
d. The amount of the note payable is calculated using the accounting equation, A = L + OE. Total assets can be determined based on items (a), (b), and (c); total owners' equity is known after considering item (e); and the note payable is the difference between total liabilities and the accounts payable.
e. Retained earnings represents the difference between cumulative net income and cumulative dividends.

Assets:			Liabilities and Owners' Equity:	
Cash		$ 700	Note payable	$ 2,200
Accounts receivable		3,400	Accounts payable	3,400
Land		7,000	Total liabilities	$ 5,600
Automobile	$9,000		Common stock	8,000
Less: Accumulated depreciation	(3,000)	6,000	Retained earnings	3,500
			Total owners' equity	11,500
Total assets		$17,100	Total liabilities and owners' equity	$17,100

P2-21.

OPTICO, INC.
Balance Sheet
December 31, 2002

Assets			Liabilities		
Current assets:			Current liabilities:		
Cash		$ 10,000	Short-term debt	$	0
Accounts receivable		10,000	Accounts payable		20,000
Merchandise inventory		45,000	Other accrued liabilities		9,000
Total current assets		$ 65,000	Total current liabilities		$ 29,000
Plant and Equipment:			Long-term debt		39,000
Land		$ 8,000	Total liabilities		$ 68,000
Building		122,000	**Owners' Equity**		
Less: Accumulated depreciation		(51,000)	Common stock, no par		$ 10,000
Total plant and equipment		$ 79,000	Retained earnings *		66,000
			Total owners' equity		$ 76,000
Total assets		$144,000	Total liabilities and owners' equity		$144,000

* Retained earnings, 12/31/01	$41,000
Add: Net income	37,000
Less: Dividends	(12,000)
Retained earnings, 12/31/02	$66,000

P2-23. a.

	2000	*1999*
Net sales and other income............	$166,809	$139,208
Less: Other income	(1,796)	(1,574)
Net sales	$165,013	$137,634
Less: Cost of sales.	(129,664)	(108,725)
Gross profit..........	**$ 35,349**	**$ 28,909**
Gross profit/net sales................	21.42%	21.00%

The change in the gross profit/net sales ratio during the year ended January 31, 2000 was insignificant, suggesting that Wal-Mart's sales mix and pricing strategies have been consistent

b.

	2000	*1999*
Gross profit (from part *a* above)...	$ 35,349	$ 28,909
Operating, selling, and general and administrative expenses	(27,040)	(22,363)
Operating income..	**$ 8,309**	**$ 6,546**
Operating income/net sales...........	5.04%	4.76%

The change in operating income as a percentage of net sales during the fiscal year ended on January 31, 2000 was slightly favorable, due primarily to the increase in gross profit margin (as calculated in part *a)* which carried through to increase operating income.

c.

	2000	*1999*
Operating income (from part *b* above)	$ 8,309	$ 6,546
Other income	1,796	1,574
Interest costs........	(1,022)	(797)
Other non-operating expenses	(368)	(153)
Income before taxes	$ 8,715	$ 7,170
Provision for income taxes	(3,338)	(2,740)
Net income	$ 5,377	$ 4,430

Solution approach: The key to answering part *c* correctly is to recast the income statement data as shown above, remembering to include "Other income" as a source of non-operating revenue. The "Income before taxes" line has been added to emphasize the importance of understanding the difference between operating and non-operating items on the income statement. The problem could be solved without calculating this number.

E3-1. a. $\quad\quad$ Amount of return $\quad\quad$ $50 $\quad\quad$ $53

$\quad\quad$ ROI = Amount invested $\quad$ Julie: $560 = **8.93%** $\quad\quad$ Sam: $620 = **8.55%**

Julie's investment is preferred because it has the higher ROI.

b. Risk is a principal factor to be considered.

E3-3. *Solution approach:* Calculate the amount of return from each alternative, then calculate the ROI of the additional return from the higher paying investment relative to the $200 that must be invested to get the higher return.

ROI * amount invested = amount of return.

Alternative # 1 $\quad$ 10% $\;*\;$ $500 = **$50 return.**
Alternative # 2 $\quad$ 11% $\;*\;$ $700 = **$77 return.**

The extra amount of return of $27 on an additional investment of $200 is an ROI of 13.5%. **($27 / $200 = 13.5%)**. Therefore, do not pay an interest rate of more than 13.5% to borrow the additional $200 needed for the higher yield investment.

E3-5. The following model can be used to help answer any questions related to ROI:

ROI	=	MARGIN	x	TURNOVER
NET INCOME		NET INCOME		SALES
AVERAGE TOTAL ASSETS	=	SALES	x	AVERAGE TOTAL ASSETS

a. 18% ROI = 12% Margin * ($600,000 Sales / Average total assets)
Average total assets = **$400,000**

b. ROI = ($78,000 Net income / $950,000 Average total assets) = **8.21%**

1.3 Turnover = (Sales / $950,000 Average total assets)
$\quad\quad$ Sales = **$1,235,000**

Margin = ($78,000 Net income / $1,235,000 Sales) = **6.32%**

ROI = (6.32% Margin * 1.3 Turnover) = 8.21%

c. 7.37% ROI = (Margin * 2.1 Turnover)
$\quad$ Margin = **3.5%**

E3-7.   Remember that "net assets" is the same as "owners' equity."

Beginning net assets.	$346,800
Add: Net income......	42,300
Less: Dividends........	(12,000)
Ending net assets......	$377,100

ROE = Net income / Average owners' equity
    = $42,300 / (($346,800 + $377,100) / 2) = **11.7%**

E3-9. a.

	Do Not Prepay Accounts Payable	Prepay Accounts Payable
Current assets.....	$ 12,639	$ 8,789
- Current liabilities	(7,480)	(3,630)
= Working capital..	$ 5,159	$ 5,159
Current ratio	1.69	2.42

Payment of the accounts payable does not affect working capital, but does improve the current ratio. Is this balance sheet "window dressing" worth the opportunity cost of not being able to invest the cash? Remember, once the payment is made, the cash is in someone else's hands.

b.

	Without Loan	With Loan
Current assets.....	$ 12,639	$ 17,639
- Current liabilities.	(7,480)	(12,480)
= Working capital..	$ 5,159	$ 5,159
= Current ratio	1.69	1.41

If the loan is taken after the end of the fiscal year, the current ratio on the year-end balance sheet will be higher than if the loan is taken before the end of the year. Working capital is not affected. Thus, it makes sense to wait until after the end of the year to borrow on a short-term basis, unless cash is needed immediately.

P3-11. a. ROI = Margin * Turnover
    = (Net income / Net revenues) * (Net revenues / Average total assets)
    = ($7,314 / $29,389) * ($29,389 / (($31,471 + $43,849) / 2))
    = (24.9% Margin * 0.78 Turnover) = **19.4%**

b. ROE = Net income / Average stockholders' equity
    = $7,314 / (($23,377 + $32,535) / 2) = **26.2%**

3-11. c. Working capital = Current assets - Current liabilities

	12/25/99	*12/26/98*
Current assets.....	$17,819	$13,475
- Current liabilities	(7,099)	(5,804)
= Working capital..	**$10,720**	**$ 7,671**

d. Current ratio = Current assets / Current liabilities

	12/25/99	*12/26/98*
Current assets.....	$17,819	$13,475
/ Current liabilities	(7,099)	(5,804)
= Current ratio	**2.51**	**2.32**

e. Acid-test ratio = (Cash + Short-term securities + Accounts and Notes receivable)
                     Current liabilities

	12/25/99	*12/26/98*
Cash and cash equivalents	$ 3,695	$ 2,038
Short-term investments.............	7,705	5,272
Trading assets	388	316
Accounts receivable, net............	3,700	3,527
Total (quick assets)	$15,488	$11,153
Total (quick assets)	$15,488	$11,153
/ Current liabilities	7,099	5,804
= Acid-test ratio	**2.18**	**1.92**

P3-13. a. Working capital = Current assets - Current liabilities

	1/31/02	*1/31/01*
Current assets.......	$ 14	$ 18
- Current liabilities....	(9)	(6)
= Working capital.....	**$ 5**	**$ 12**

Current ratio = Current assets / Current liabilities

	1/31/02	*1/31/01*
Current assets.......	$ 14	$ 18
/ Current liabilities...	9	6
= Current ratio	**1.56**	**3.0**

b. Even though the firm has more cash at January 31, 2002, it is less liquid based on the working capital and current ratio measures. The firm owes more on accounts payable, and has less inventory to sell and fewer accounts receivable to collect, as compared to January 31, 2001.

P3-13. c. Accounts receivable were collected, inventories were reduced, and current liabilities increased. These changes and the increase in cash are all possible, because changes in a firm's cash position and its profitability are not directly related.

P3-15. a. 15% ROI = (Margin * 2.0 Turnover)
Margin required as a manufacturer = **7.5%**

2.0 Turnover = (Sales / $6,000,000 Average total assets)
Sales required as a manufacturer = **$12,000,000**

7.5% Margin = (Net Income / $12,000,000 Sales)
Net Income required as a manufacturer = **$900,000** (or $0.9 million)

b. 15% ROI = (Net Income / $1,000,000 Average total assets)
Net Income required as a service firm = **$150,000**

15% ROI = (2.5% Margin * Turnover)
Turnover required as a service firm = **6.0**

6.0 Turnover = (Sales / $1,000,000 Average total assets)
Sales required as a service firm = **$6,000,000** (or $6 million)

The Bookkeeping Process and Transaction Analysis

E4-1.

Trans-action	Cash	Accounts Receivable	Supplies	Equipment	Notes Payable	Accounts Payable	Paid in Capital	Revenues	Expenses
	ASSETS				**= LIABILITIES +**		**OWNERS' EQUITY**		
a.	+8,000						+8,000		
b.	+5,000				+5,000				
c.	-1,750			+1,750					
d.	-1,400								-1,400
e.	-9,000		+15,000			+6,000			
f.	+6,500		-4,000					+6,500	-4,000
g.						+100			-100
h.	-1,200		+4,200			+3,000			
i.	+3,900	+9,600	-9,000					+13,500	-9,000
j.						+1,850*			-1,850
k.	+3,160	-3,160							
l.	-4,720					-4,720			
	8,490 +	6,440 +	6,200 +	1,750 =	5,000 +	6,230 +	8,000 +	20,000 -	16,350

Month-end totals: **Assets $22,880 = Liabilities $11,230 + Owners' equity $11,650**

Net income for the month: **Revenues $20,000 - Expenses $16,350 = Net income $3,650**

* Ordinarily, the Wages Payable account would be increased for employee wage expense that has been incurred but not yet paid.

Optional Continuation:

BLUE CO. STORES, INC.
Income Statement

Sales	$20,000
Cost of goods sold	(13,000)
Gross profit...	$ 7,000
Rent expense.	(1,400)
Wages expense.........	(1,850)
Advertising expense	(100)
Net income (this exercise ignores income taxes)	$ 3,650

E4-1. *(continued)*

BLUE CO. STORES, INC.
Balance Sheet

Assets:

Cash	$ 8,490
Accounts receivable	6,440
Merchandise inventory	6,200
Total current assets	$21,130
Equipment (this exercise ignores depreciation)	1,750
Total assets	$22,880

Liabilities:

Notes payable..........	$ 5,000
Accounts payable	6,230
Total liabilities..........	$11,230

Owners' Equity:

Paid-in Capital..........	$ 8,000
Retained earnings.....	3,650
Total owners' equity	$11,650
Total liabilities and owners' equity...	$22,880

* Since this was the first month of operations, the Retained Earnings account would have a $0 beginning balance. Thus, the net income for the month creates a positive balance in retained earnings.

E4-3. a. Dr. Cash .. .. $ 8,000

     Cr. Paid-In Capital .... $ 8,000

   b. Dr. Cash.....   5,000

     Cr. Note Payable..........   5,000

   c. Dr. Equipment.......   1,750

     Cr. Cash..........   1,750

   d. Dr. Rent Expense   1,400

     Cr. Cash..........   1,400

   e. Dr. Merchandise Inventory   15,000

     Cr. Cash..........   9,000

     Cr. Accounts Payable   6,000

E4-3. f. Dr. Cash.. 6,500
  Cr. Sales Revenue 6,500
  Dr. Cost of Goods Sold... 4,000
  Cr. Merchandise Inventory 4,000

g. Dr. Advertising Expense.. 100
  Cr. Accounts Payable 100

h. Dr. Merchandise Inventory... 4,200
  Cr. Cash 1,200
  Cr. Accounts Payable 3,000

i. Dr. Cash... 3,900
  Dr. Accounts Receivable 9,600
  Cr. Sales Revenue 13,500
  Dr. Cost of Goods Sold 9,000
  Cr. Merchandise Inventory 9,000

j. Dr. Wages Expense 1,850
  Cr. Accounts (or Wages) Payable 1,850

k. Dr. Cash.. 3,160
  Cr. Accounts Receivable 3,160

l. Dr. Accounts Payable 4,720
  Cr. Cash... 4,720

E4-5.

Transaction/Situation	*A*	*=*	*L*	*+*	*OE*	*Net Income*
a. Example transaction.	Supplies -1,400					Supplies Exp -1,400
b. Paid an insurance premium of $480 for the coming year. An asset, prepaid insurance, was debited	Prepaid Insurance +480 Cash -480					
c. Paid $3,200 of wages for the current month	Cash -3,200					Wages Exp -3,200

E4-5. *Transaction/Situation*	*A*	*=*	*L*	*+*	*OE*	*Net Income*
d. Received $250 of interest income for the current month	Cash +250					Interest Inc +250
e. Accrued $700 of commissions payable to sales staff for the current month ...			Commissions Payable +700			Commissions Expense −700
f. Accrued $130 of interest expense at the end of the month.....................			Interest Pay +130			Interest Exp −130
g. Received $2,100 on accounts receivable accrued at the end of the prior month	Cash +2,100 Accounts Rec −2,100					
h. Purchased $600 of merchandise inventory from a supplier on account	Merch Inventory +600		Accounts Payable +600			
i. Paid $160 of interest expense for the month......	Cash −160					Interest Exp −160
j. Accrued $800 of wages at the end of the current month..			Wages Pay +800			Wages Exp −800
k. Paid $500 of accounts payable.........	Cash −500		Accounts Pay −500			

E4-5.			
a. Dr. Supplies Expense.....................	$1,400	
Cr. Supplies		$1,400
b. Dr. Prepaid Insurance.....................	480	
Cr. Cash...........		480
c. Dr. Wages Expense	3,200	
Cr. Cash...........		3,200
d. Dr. Cash......	250	
Cr. Interest Income		250

E4-5. e. Dr. Commissions Expense............ .... $ 700
         Cr. Commissions Payable .... $ 700

    f. Dr. Interest Expense   130
         Cr. Interest Payable   130

    g. Dr. Cash   2,100
         Cr. Accounts Receivable   2,100

    h. Dr. Merchandise Inventory............   600
         Cr. Accounts Payable   600

    i. Dr. Interest Expense   160
         Cr. Cash..........   160

    j. Dr. Wages Expense   800
         Cr. Wages Payable   800

    k. Dr. Accounts Payable   500
         Cr. Cash..........   500

E4-7.

Transaction/Situation	*A*	*=*	*L*	*+*	*OE*	*Net Income*
a. Example transaction	+550					+550
b. Paid an insurance premium of $360 for the coming year. An asset, "prepaid insurance" was debited	-360 +360					
c. Recognized insurance for one month from the above premium via a reclassification adjusting entry	-30					-30
d. Paid $800 of wages accrued at the end of the prior month......................	-800		-800			
e. Paid $2,600 of wages for the current month	-2,600					-2,600
f. Accrued $600 of wages at the end of the current month..			+600			-600
g. Received cash of $1,500 on accounts receivable accrued in prior month.....	+1,500 -1,500					

E4-7. a. Dr. Accounts Receivable................. .... $ 550
        Cr. Service Revenue .... $ 550

   b. Dr. Prepaid Insurance..................   360
        Cr. Cash...........   360

   c. Dr. Insurance Expense.................   30
        Cr. Prepaid Insurance   30

   d. Dr. Wages Payable   800
        Cr. Cash........   800

   e. Dr. Wages Expense.   2,600
        Cr. Cash   2,600

   f. Dr. Wages Expense.   600
        Cr. Wages Payable   600

   g. Dr. Cash   1,500
        Cr. Accounts Receivable   1,500

E4-9. Prepare an analysis of the change in stockholders' equity for the month, showing the effects of the net loss and dividends:

Balance, February 1, 2002................. .... $ 630,000
Revenues........ .... $123,000
Expenses........ ....   (131,000)   (8,000)
Dividends....... ....   (12,000)
Balance, February 28, 2002................ ....   **$ 610,000**

E4-11. a. *4/1/2002*
        Dr. Note Receivable $6,000
            Cr. Accounts Receivable $6,000

    b. *12/31/2002*
        Dr. Interest Receivable.............   675
            Cr. Interest Revenue ($6,000 * 15% * 9/12)   675

E4-11. c. *3/31/2003*

Dr. Cash.	6,900	
Cr. Note Receivable		6,000
Cr. Interest Receivable		675
Cr. Interest Revenue............		225

In entry *c*, only $675 of the total interest of $900 had been accrued, so the Interest Receivable account is reduced by the $675 that had been accrued in 2002; the other $225 that is received is recorded as interest revenue for 2003, the year in which it was earned.

Balance Sheet		Income Statement
Assets = Liabilities + Owners' Equity	**← Net income = Revenues - Expenses**	

a. *Receipt of note on April 1, 2002*:
Notes Receivable
+6,000
Account Receivable
-6,000

b. *Accrual of 9 month's interest at December 31, 2002*:

Interest Receivable +675		Interest Revenue +675

Balance Sheet		Income Statement
Assets = Liabilities + Owners' Equity	**← Net income = Revenues - Expenses**	

c. *Collection of note and interest at March 31, 2003*:
Cash
+6,900
Note Receivable
-6,000
Interest Receivable
-675

Interest
Revenue
+225

E4-13. a. Net income for October would be overstated, because an expense was not recorded.

b. Net income for November would be understated, because November expenses would include an expense from October.

c. There wouldn't be any effect on net income for the two months combined, because the overstatement and understatement offset.

d. To match revenues and expenses, which results in more accurate financial statements.

E4-15. a. $1,200 + ? - $1,500 = $2,100$. Thus, the February 28 adjustment = **$2,400**

    b. The Cash account would most likely have been credited for the amount of the February transactions, and would represent the payment of previously accrued interest.

    c. The Interest Expense account would most likely have been debited for the February adjustment, and would represent the accrual of interest expense for February.

    d. The entry would have been made to make the income statement and balance sheet more accurate. The adjusting entry resulted in a better matching of revenue and expense for February.

P4-17. a. Dr. Cash.. $1,000,000

         Cr. Common Stock $1,000,000

    b. Dr. Cash.. 500,000

         Cr. Notes Payable.. 500,000

    c. Dr. Salaries Expense 380,000

         Cr. Cash.. 380,000

    d. Dr. Merchandise Inventory...................................... 640,000

         Cr. Accounts Payable 640,000

    e. Dr. Accounts Receivable 910,000

         Cr. Sales 910,000

      Dr. Cost of Goods Sold... 580,000

         Cr. Merchandise Inventory 580,000

    f. Dr. Rent Expense.. 110,000

         Cr. Cash.. 110,000

    g. Dr. Equipment.. 150,000

         Cr. Cash.. 50,000

         Cr. Accounts Payable 100,000

    h. Dr. Accounts Payable 720,000

         Cr. Cash.. 720,000

    i. Dr. Utilities Expense 36,000

         Cr. Cash.. 36,000

P4-17. j. Dr. Cash $825,000

       Cr. Accounts Receivable $825,000

k. Dr. Interest Expense 60,000

      Cr. Interest Payable.................   60,000

l. Dr. Rent Expense 10,000

      Cr. Rent Payable (or Accounts Payable)   10,000

Balance Sheet			Income Statement		
Assets = Liabilities + Owners' Equity			**← Net income = Revenues - Expenses**		
a. Cash	Common Stock				
+1,000,000	+1,000,000				
b. Cash	Notes Payable *LT*				
+500,000	+500,000 *loan*				
c. Cash					Salaries Exp
-380,000					-380,000
d. Merchandise	Accounts				
Inventory	Payable *Accounts Pay*				
+640,000	+640,000				
e. Accounts Rec				Sales	
+910,000				+910,000	Cost of
Merchandise Inv					Goods Sold
-580,000					-580,000
f. Cash					Rent Exp
-110,000					-110,000
g. Equipment	Accounts				
+150,000	Payable *Accounts Pay*				
Cash	+100,000				
-50,000					
h. Cash	Accounts				
-720,000	Payable *Accounts Pay*				
	-720,000				

P4-17.	Balance Sheet			Income Statement		
	Assets	= Liabilities	+ Owners' Equity	← Net income	= Revenues	- Expenses
i.	Cash -36,000					Utilities Exp -36,000
j.	Cash +825,000 Accounts Rec -825,000					
k.		Interest Pay +60,000				Interest Exp -60,000
l.		Rent Payable +10,000				Rent Exp -10,000

P4-19. a.

Net sales	$741,000
Cost of goods sold	(329,000)
Gross profit..	412,000
General and administrative expenses	(83,000)
Advertising expense	(76,000)
Other selling expenses	(42,000)
Income from operations (operating income)	**$211,000**

b.

Income from operations (operating income)...........................	$211,000
Income tax expense	(83,000)
Income before extraordinary items	128,000
Extraordinary loss from earthquake, net of tax savings of $25,000..........	(61,000)
Net income	**$ 67,000**

P4-21. a. *1/10/02*

Dr.   Paper Napkin Expense (or Supplies Expense)........... .... $4,800

     Cr.   Cash........ .... $4,800

<small>To record as an expense the cost of paper napkins purchased for cash.</small>

b. *1/31/02*

Dr.   Paper Napkins on Hand (or Supplies)...................   3,850

     Cr.   Paper Napkin Expense (or Supplies Expense)...   3,850

<small>To remove from the expense account and set up as an asset the cost
of paper napkins on hand January 31.</small>

P4-21. c. *1/10/02*

      Dr. Paper Napkins on Hand (or Supplies)............ .... $4,800

          Cr. Cash $4,800

          To set up as an asset the cost of paper napkins purchased for cash.

    d. *1/31/02*

      Dr. Paper Napkin Expense (or Supplies Expense)...........   950

          Cr.   Paper Napkins on Hand . (or Supplies)   950

          To record the cost of paper napkins used in January.

Balance Sheet	Income Statement
Assets = Liabilities + Owners' Equity	← **Net income = Revenues - Expenses**

a. *1/10/02. Record as an expense the cost of paper napkins purchased for cash:*

Cash   Supplies

-4,800   Expense

                                          -4,800

b. *1/31/02. Remove from the expense account and set up as an asset the cost of the paper napkins on hand January 31.*

Supplies   Supplies

+3,850   *(Note: A reduction in*   Expense

                   Supplies Expense.)   +3,850

c. *1/10/02. Set up as an asset the cost of paper napkins purchased for cash.*

Supplies

+4,800

Cash

-4,800

d. *1/31/02. Record the cost of paper napkins used in January.*

Supplies   Supplies

-950   Expense

                                         -950

e. Each approach results in the same expense for January ($950) and the same asset amount ($3,850) reported on the January 31 balance sheet.

P4-23. *Note:* *The key to this problem is for students to see that transactions have a direct effect on the financial statements.* To answer the questions in part *b*, students should be thinking about how Intel would record each of the transactions. To answer the questions in part *c*, students should be solving for the missing amounts in T-accounts for inventories, accounts receivable, and accounts payable.

	Assets			Liabilities	Revenues	Expenses	
	Cash and Cash Equivalents	Accounts Receivable, net	Inventories	Accounts Payable	Net Revenues	Cost of Sales	Marketing, General and Administrative Expenses
a. Beginning balance		3,527	1,582	1,244			
b. Net revenues.........		+29,839			+29,839		
Cost of sales.........			-11,836			-11,836	
Marketing, general and administrative expenses ...				+3,872			-3,872
c. Purchases of inventory on account.........			+11,732	+11,732			
Collections of accounts receivable	+29,666	-29,666					
Payment of accounts payable	-15,478			-15,478			
Ending balance.....	$ 3,700		$ 1,478	$ 1,370			

E5-1.

Balance per bank	$373	Balance per books.	$844
Less: Outstanding checks		Less: NSF check	(75)
($13 + $50).	(63)	Error in recording check	
Add: Deposit in transit	450	(as $56 instead of $65).	(9)
Reconciled balance.....	$760	Reconciled balance.........	$760

E5-3. a. Dr. Accounts Receivable *(for NSF check)* $75
 Dr. Expense (or other account originally debited *for error*) 9
  Cr. Cash.......... .... $84

Balance Sheet	Income Statement
Assets = Liabilities + Owners' Equity ← **Net income = Revenues - Expenses**	
Accounts	Expense
Receivable	(or other
+75	account)
Cash	-9
-84	

b. The cash amount to be shown on the balance sheet is the $760 reconciled amount.

E5-5.   **Allowance for Bad Debts**

Bad debt write-offs		1/1/02 balance	$13,400
(from 1/1 to 11/30)	?	Bad debt expense	
		(from 1/1 to 11/30)	21,462
		1/30/02 balance......	$ 9,763
Adjustment required (11/30/02).	?		
		12/31/02 balance....	$ 9,500

a. *Solution approach*: The bad debt write-offs from January through November can be determined by subtracting the November 30 balance from the total of the beginning balance and the bad debts expense recognized for the first 11 months.

Bad debt write-offs = $13,400 + $21,462 - $9,763 = **$25,099**

E5-5. b. The adjustment required at December 31, 2002 can be determined by comparing the November 30 balance in the allowance account to the desired ending balance.

Bad debt expense adjustment = $9,763 - $9,500 = **$263**

Dr.   Allowance for Bad Debts $263
    Cr.   Bad Debts Expense $263
To adjust the allowance account to the appropriate balance, and to correct the overstatement of expense recorded in the January through November period.

Balance Sheet		Income Statement	
Assets = Liabilities + Owners' Equity ← Net income = Revenues - Expenses			
Allowance	*(Note: A reduction in an expense increases net*		Bad Debts
for Bad Debts	*income, and a reduction in a contra-asset account*		Expense
+263	*increases total assets.)*		+263

c. The write-off will not have any effect on 2002 net income, because the write-off decreases both the accounts receivable asset and the allowance account contra-asset for equal amounts. Net income was affected when the expense was recognized.

E5-7. a. 2% * $340,000,000 * 90% = **$6,120,000,** or $6.12 million.

b. By paying within 10 days instead of 30 days, the customers are "investing" funds for 20 days, and receiving slightly more than a 2 percent return on their investment (for a $100 obligation, the return is $2 on an investment of $98). But ROI is expressed as an annual percentage rate, and there are slightly more than 18 twenty-day periods in a year. Thus the annual ROI is a little greater than 36 percent. *(See Business in Practice—Cash Discounts.)*

E5-9. a.

4 ½ months		5 ½ months	
6/15	10/31		4/15
(date of note)	*(year-end)*		*(maturity date)*

Interest earned = $4,500 principal * 13.8% rate * 4½/12 time = **$232.88**

Dr.   Interest Receivable................. .... $232.88
    Cr.   Interest Revenue............. .... $232.88
To accrue interest earned on a short-term note.

E5-9. a. *(continued)*

Balance Sheet			Income Statement		
Assets = **Liabilities** + **Owners' Equity**			← **Net income** = **Revenues** - **Expenses**		
Interest				Interest	
Receivable				Revenue	
+232.88				+232.88	

b. ***Solution approach***: What accounts are affected, and how are they affected? Cash is being received for note principal and 10 month's interest. Notes receivable is reduced because the note is being paid off. Interest receivable accrued at 10/31 is being collected. Interest revenue for 5 ½ months from 10/31 to 4/15 has been earned.

Dr. Cash ($4,500 + ($4,500 * 13.8% * 10/12)) $5,017.50
    Cr. Note Receivable $4,500.00
    Cr. Interest Receivable (accrued at 10/31).... ....   232.88
    Cr. Interest Revenue ($4,500 * 13.8% * 5 ½ /12)...... ....   284.62
    <small>To record the collection of principal and interest at the maturity date of a short-term note (for which some interest had been previously accrued).</small>

Balance Sheet			Income Statement		
Assets = **Liabilities** + **Owners' Equity**			← **Net income** = **Revenues** - **Expenses**		
Cash				Interest	
+5,017.50				Revenue	
Note Receivable				+284.62	
-4,500					
Interest Receivable					
-232.88					

E5-11. a. Under LIFO, the most recent purchase costs are released to cost of goods sold. If the *purchase cost* of inventory items is changing, the *selling price* of these same items is likely to be changing in the same direction. Thus, releasing the most recent purchase costs to the Cost of Goods Sold account results in better matching of revenue and expense.

b. During periods of rising prices, LIFO results in a balance sheet valuation that is lower than current cost. This is considered consistent with the "original cost" concept usually used to record asset values. However, it understates the "value" of inventory items because it does not reflect the current cost of inventory items. The ending inventory under FIFO more accurately reflects the value of inventory items.

E5-13. a. *March 1*

Dr. Prepaid Insurance............... .... $3,000
Cr. Cash........ .... $3,000
  To record the payment of a one-year insurance premium.

Balance Sheet			Income Statement		
Assets = **Liabilities** + **Owners' Equity**		←	**Net income** = **Revenues** - **Expenses**		
Prepaid Insurance					
+3,000					
Cash -3,000					

b. *Each month-end*:

Dr. Insurance Expense.................. .... $250
Cr. Prepaid Insurance............. .... $250
  To record the expiration of prepaid insurance each month.

Balance Sheet			Income Statement		
Assets = **Liabilities** + **Owners' Equity**		←	**Net income** = **Revenues** - **Expenses**		
Prepaid Insurance					Insurance Exp.
-250					-250

c. At August 31, 6 months of insurance coverage has been used, and 6 months is still to be used. So one-half of the original premium of $3,000, or $1,500 is prepaid and will be shown on the August 31 balance sheet as a current asset.

d. The prepaid amount is $4,500, for coverage for the 18 months. Only $3,000 of this amount is a current asset, because of the one-year time frame for current assets. Thus, $1,500 of the prepaid amount is technically a noncurrent asset.

e. To result in better matching of revenues and expenses, and a more meaningful net income amount. Although the expenditure of cash has been made, the item relates to the earning of revenue in a subsequent accounting period.

E5-15.

	Current Assets	*Current Liabilities*	*Owners' Equity*	*Net Income*
b. Determined that the Allowance for Bad Debts balance should be increased by $2,200.	Allowance for Bad Debts -2,200			Bad Debts Expense -2,200

E5-15.

	Current Assets	Current Liabilities	Owners' Equity	Net Income
c. Recognized bank service $30 for the month.	Cash -30			Service Charge Exp. -30
d. Received $25 cash for interest receivable that had been accrued in a prior month.	Cash +25 Interest Receivable -25			
e. Purchased five units of a new item of inventory on account at a cost of $35 each.	Inventory +175	Accounts Payable +175		
f. Purchased 10 more units of the above item at a cost of $38 each.	Inventory +380	Accounts Payable * +380		

* Could also be recorded as: Cash -380 under the current assets category.

	Current Assets			Net Income
g. Sold eight of the items purchased (in *e* and *f* above), and recognized the cost of goods sold using the FIFO cost-flow assumption.	Inventory -289 *(5 units @ $35, 3 units @ $38)*			Cost of Goods Sold -289

E5-17.

	Current Assets	Current Liabilities	Owners' Equity	Net Income
b. Recorded estimated bad debts in the amount of $700.	Allowance for Bad Debts -700			Bad Debts Expense -700
c. Wrote off an overdue account receivable of $520.	Accounts Receivable -520 Allowance for Doubtful Accounts +520			*(Net realizable value of accounts receivable is not affected.)*

E5-17.

	Current Assets	Current Liabilities	Owners' Equity	Net Income
d. Converted a customer's $1,200 overdue account receivable into a note.	Notes Receivable +1,200 Accounts Receivable -1,200			
e. Accrued $48 of interest earned on the note (in *d* above).	Interest Receivable +48			Interest Revenue +48
f. Collected the accrued interest (in *e* above).	Cash +48 Interest Receivable -48			
g. Recorded $4,000 of sales, 80% of which were on account.	Cash +800 Accounts Receivable +3,200			Sales +4,000
h. Recognized cost of goods sold in the amount of $3,200.	Inventory -3,200			Cost of Goods Sold -3,200

P5-19. **Solution approach:** Set up a bank reconciliation in the usual format, enter the known information, and then work backwards to solve for the beginning balances in the company's Cash account and on the bank statement (these are referred to as the "Indicated balance" amounts in Exhibit 5-2 in the text).

Indicated balance (per bank)... $?		Indicated balance (per books)......	$?
Less: Outstanding checks .... (3,000)		Less: NSF check	(400)
Add: Deposits in transit.......... 2,100		Bank service charge........	(50)
		Add: Check recording error........	90
Reconciled balance..... .... $4,800		Reconciled balance........	$4,800

P5-19. *(continued)*

Key: To solve for the beginning (i.e., indicated) balances, the effects of reconciling items must be reversed out of the known ending (i.e., reconciled) balances.

a. Balance per Cash account before reconciliation = $4,800 - 90 + 400 + 50 = **$5,160**

b. Balance per bank before reconciliation = $4,800 - 2,100 + 3,000 = **$5,700**

P5-21. a.   **Allowance for Bad Debts**

Bad debt write-offs (during the year) $11,800	12/31/01 balance $17,900
	Bad debt expense .. .. ?
	12/31/02 balance ... . $ 9,500

Bad debt expense = $11,800 - $17,900 + $9,500 = **$3,400**

b. 1. Working capital would not be affected because the write-off entry decreases both the accounts receivable asset and the allowance account contra-asset by equal amounts.

   Dr.   Allowance for Bad Debts $3,100
       Cr.   Accounts Receivable $3,100
   To write off a past due account as uncollectible.

Balance Sheet			Income Statement	
Assets =	**Liabilities** +	**Owners' Equity**	← **Net income** =	**Revenues** - **Expenses**
Accounts Receivable -3,100				
Allowance for Bad Debts +3,100				

2. Net income would not be affected by the write-off entry because it does not adjust any expense or revenue accounts. ROI would not be affected because net income and total assets are not changed.

c. Sales were *probably* lower in 2002 because the accounts receivable balance has decreased during the year—but this cannot be determined for sure without information about the cash collections of accounts receivable.

P5-23. ***Solution approach:*** Net realizable value = Accounts receivable - Allowance for bad debts. The balance sheet presentation of this information at December 31, 2002 (ending balances) is provided with the problem information. Your task is to work backwards to determine the balances in these accounts at December 31, 2001 (beginning balances).

Accounts Receivable

12/31/01 balance......	$?		Cash collections..	$410,000
Sales on account	400,000		Accounts written off.......	15,000
12/31/02 balance......	$ 50,000			

December 31, 2001 balance = $410,000 + $15,000 - $400,000 + $50,000 = **$75,000.** This makes sense because the credits to accounts receivable during the year for cash collections and write-offs exceeded the debit for sales on account.

Allowance for Bad Debts

Bad debt write-offs			12/31/01 balance.....	$?
(during the year)..	$15,000		Bad debt expense....	12,000
			12/31/02 balance.....	$ 7,000

December 31, 2001 balance = $7,000 + $15,000 - $12,000 = **$10,000.** This makes sense because Carr Co. wrote-off more accounts during the year than it added to the allowance account with the bad debts expense adjustment.

> ***At December 31, 2001:***
> Accounts receivable $75,000
> Less: Allowance for bad debts.... .... (10,000) $65,000

P5-25. a. ***Ending inventory calculations:***

	--------- FIFO ----------	--------- LIFO ----------
Blowers........	10 of 11/7 @ 200 = $2,000	10 of 1/21 @ 200 = $2,000
Mowers........	20 of 9/20 @ 210 = $4,200	20 of 4/6 @ 210 = $4,200
	5 of 8/15 @ 215 = 1,075	5 of 5/22 @ 215 = 1,075
	$5,275	$5,275

P5-25. a. *(continued)*

> *Analysis of results:* In this problem, there is no difference between ending inventories, and therefore there won't be any difference between cost of goods sold under either alternative. Neither the amount of goods available for sale (the sum of the beginning inventory and purchases amounts) nor the amount of ending inventory are affected by the inventory cost flow assumption used. Why? Look carefully at the cost per unit of inventory items that were purchased during the year. Notice that the costs per unit of the beginning inventory and the cost per unit of items purchased on September 20 and November 7 are the same.

> b. Probably LIFO, because the higher cost of the most recent (last-in) purchase will become part of the cost of goods sold, thus increasing cost, decreasing profits, and decreasing the firm's income tax obligation.

P5-27. *Solution approach*: Calculate goods available for sale in units and dollars, and ending inventory in units. These amounts are the same for both FIFO and LIFO under either a periodic or a perpetual inventory system.

```
Beginning inventory.....................   150 @ $30 =   $ 4,500
Purchases...............................    70 @   33 =     2,310
                                            90 @   35 =     3,150
                                           140 @   36 =     5,040
                                            50 @   38 =     1,900
Goods available for sale ...............   500             $16,900
Sales...................................  (300)
Ending inventory........................   200 units

a. FIFO periodic cost of goods sold ....   150 @ $30 =   $ 4,500
                                            70 @   33 =     2,310
                                            80 @   35 =     2,800
                                                         $ 9,610

   FIFO periodic ending inventory.......    10 @   35 =   $   350
                                           140 @   36 =     5,040
                                            50 @   38 =     1,900
                                                         $ 7,290
                                                          $16,900

   LIFO periodic cost of goods sold.....    50 @ $38 =   $ 1,900
                                           140 @   36 =     5,040
                                            90 @   35 =     3,150
                                            20 @   33 =       660
                                                          $10,750
```

P5-27. a. *(continued)*

```
LIFO periodic ending inventory................    150 @  30 =  $ 4,500
                                                   50 @  33 =    1,650
                                                                $ 6,150
                                                                $16,900
```

b. FIFO perpetual cost of goods sold........

```
                               3/7 sale 100 @ $30 = $ 3,000
                               9/28 sale  50 @  30 =   1,500
                                          50 @  33 =   1,650
                               12/4 sale  20 @  33 =     660
                                          80 @  35 =   2,800
                                                     $ 9,610
```

FIFO perpetual ending inventory..........

```
                                10 @  35 = $    350
                               140 @  36 =    5,040
                                50 @  38 =    1,900
                                          $ 7,290
                                          $16,900
```

LIFO perpetual cost of goods sold........

```
                               3/7 sale   70 @ $33 = $ 2,310
                                          30 @  30 =     900
                               9/28 sale 100 @  36 =   3,600.
                               12/4 sale  50 @  38 =   1,900
                                          40 @  36 =   1,440
                                          10 @  35 =     350
                                                     $10,500
```

LIFO perpetual ending inventory..........

```
                               120 @ 30 = $ 3,600
                                80 @ 35 =   2,800
                                          $ 6,400
                                          $16,900
```

c. Under FIFO, the periodic and perpetual inventory systems *always* result in the same dollar amounts being assigned to ending inventory and cost of goods sold—once first-in, always first-in—and the timing of the application of the FIFO rules makes no difference. Under LIFO, the "last-in cost" changes each time another inventory item is purchased. Thus, the timing of the application of the LIFO rules is relevant, and different results will occur under the periodic and perpetual systems. These relationships are discussed in the Business in Practice—The Perpetual Inventory System.

P5-29. a.

Inventory		Cost of Goods Sold	
Balance is $5,000 too high	Credit to correct error	Debit to correct inventory error	

To correct the overstatement, inventory should be reduced (credited) $5,000, and cost of goods sold should be increased (debited) $5,000. If the error is not corrected, cost of goods sold will be too low and net income will be too high.

b. If ending inventory were understated (too low) cost of goods sold would be overstated (too high) and net income would be understated (too low).

Accounting for and Presentation of Property, Plant and Equipment, and Other Noncurrent Assets

E6-1. a. Allocate the purchase cost in proportion to appraised values.

Cost of land = ($20,000 / ($80,000 + $20,000)) * $90,000 = **$18,000**

b. Land is not a depreciable asset. Management would want as much of the purchase price as feasible to be assigned to assets whose cost will become a tax-deductible expense in future years--reducing taxable income and income taxes payable.

c. All ordinary and necessary costs incurred by Dorsey Co. in order to get the land ready for its intended use should be added to the Land account. Thus, the cost included in the Land account is the total amount paid, plus the cost of razing building. Note that no costs are added to Dorsey Co.'s Buildings account because the building was not acquired with the intent to be used as a building.

Cost of land = $90,000 + $10,000 = **$100,000**

d. Appraised values are be used because they represent the *current* asset values (at the time of purchase by Dorsey Co.). The old original cost data represent what the relative asset values were (at the time of purchase by Bibb Co.), which is not relevant to Dorsey Co.

E6-3. a. Expense. Routine repair and maintenance costs would not increase the useful life or estimated salvage of the vehicles, so the "economic benefits" of these expenditures relate only to the current year.

b. Asset. The cost of developing the coal mine should be capitalized (as a natural resource) because the extraction of coal will generate revenues in future years. The $60,000 cost of developing the coal mine will be recorded as depletion expense (at a rate of six cents per ton extracted).

c. Asset. This cost should be added to the Building account because it will extend the useful life of the asset.

E6.3. d. Expense. Advertising costs are *always* treated as expenses in the year incurred because it is impossible to determine to what extent, if any, future-period revenues will be affected by current-period advertising expenditures.

e. Asset. This cost should be added to the Land account because it is an ordinary and necessary cost incurred to get the land ready for its intended use.

E6-5. Alpha, Inc. should have a higher ROI than Beta Co. Alpha, Inc.'s plant is older and will be depreciated to a greater extent than Beta Co.'s. Thus, Alpha, Inc.'s asset base will be lower, so its ROI will be higher. The implication for Beta Co. is that because of its lower ROI, its ability to raise capital will be reduced unless it has production and/or technological advantages or efficiencies.

E6-7. a. Amount to be depreciated = Cost – Salvage value
Annual depreciation expense = Amount to be depreciated / Useful life
Annual depreciation expense = ($80,000 – $8,000) / 8 = $9,000 per year
After 5 years, accumulated depreciation = $9,000 * 5 = **$45,000**

b. Straight-line rate = 1 / 8 = 12.5%. Double-declining rate = 12.5% * 2 = **25%**

Year	Net Book Value at Beginning of Year	Depreciation Expense	At End of Year Accumulated Depreciation	At End of Year Net Book Value
1	$80,000	$80,000 * 25% = $20,000	$20,000	$60,000
2	60,000	60,000 * 25% = 15,000	35,000	45,000
3	45,000	45,000 * 25% = **11,250**	46,250	33,750

c. Sum of the digits for an 8-year life = 8 + 7 + 6 + 5 + 4 + 3 + 2 + 1 = 36 digits
Amount to be depreciated = $80,000 cost – $8,000 salvage value = $72,000

Solution approach: Accumulated depreciation at the end of the fifth year equals the sum of the depreciation expense amounts recorded in the first five years.

After 5 years, accumulated depreciation = ((8 + 7 + 6 + 5 + 4) / 36) * $72,000
= (30 / 36) * $72,000 = **$60,000**

Under sum-of-the-years'-digits, accumulated depreciation after 5 years is $15,000 higher ($60,000 – $45,000), than under straight-line because of the accelerated depreciation pattern.

E6-7. d. Net book value = Cost − Accumulated depreciation. After 8 years, the asset will have been fully depreciated to its estimated salvage value of $8,000 under each method. Accumulated depreciation will be $72,000, and net book value will be $8,000 ($80,000 − $72,000).

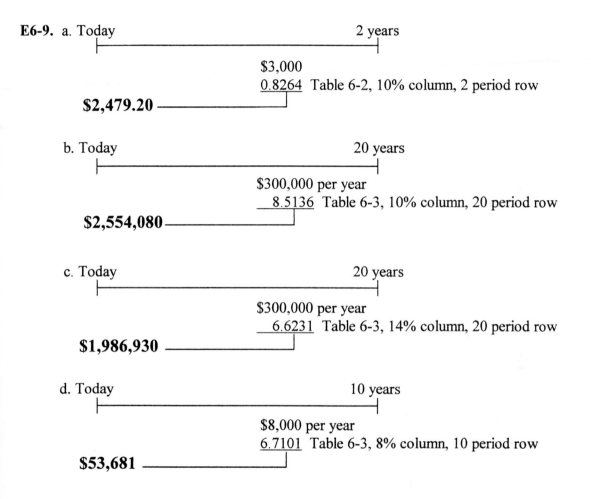

E6-9. a. Today   2 years

$3,000
0.8264   Table 6-2, 10% column, 2 period row

$2,479.20

b. Today   20 years

$300,000 per year
8.5136   Table 6-3, 10% column, 20 period row

$2,554,080

c. Today   20 years

$300,000 per year
6.6231   Table 6-3, 14% column, 20 period row

$1,986,930

d. Today   10 years

$8,000 per year
6.7101   Table 6-3, 8% column, 10 period row

$53,681

E6-11. a. Yes, because of the above-average ROI of 18%, I could afford to invest **$40,000** more than $200,000 and still earn a 15% ROI--which is the rate I'd expect to earn from an investment in this type of business. The excess earnings offered by this investment = ($200,000 * 18%) − ($200,000 * 15%) = $36,000 − $30,000 = **$6,000 per year** on a $200,000 investment. At an ROI of 15%, an investment of **$240,000** would be required to earn $36,000 of income, so that is the maximum price I'd be willing to pay for the business.

E6-11. b. Each of the individual assets acquired would be recorded at their fair market values, and $40,000 would be recorded as "Goodwill."

E6-13.	*Assets*	*Liabilities*	*Net Income*
b. Sold land that had originally cost $9,000 for $14,000 in cash.	Land – 9,000 Cash + 14,000		Gain on Sale of Land + 5,000
c. Acquired a new machine under a capital lease. The present value of future lease payments, discounted at 10%, was $12,000.	Machine + 12,000	Capital Lease Liability + 12,000	
d. Recorded the first annual payment of $2,000 for the leased machine (in c above).	Cash – 2,000	Capital Lease Liability – 800 *(Interest = $12,000 * 10%).*	Interest Expense – 1,200
e. Recorded a $6,000 payment for the cost of developing and registering a trademark.	Trademark + 6,000 Cash – 6,000		
f. Recognized the periodic amortization on the trademark (in e above) using a 40-year useful life.	Trademark – 150		Amortization Expense – 150
g. Sold used production equipment for $16,000 in cash. The equipment originally cost $40,000. The accumulated depreciation account had a balance of $22,000 before adjusting for a $1,000 year-to-date depreciation entry that must be recorded before the sale of the equipment is recorded.	Accumulated Depreciation – 1,000, + 23,000 Equipment – 40,000 Cash + 16,000		Depreciation Expense – 1,000 Loss on Sale of Equipment – 1,000

P6-15. a. Repair cost capitalized in error = $20,000.

Depreciation expense in current year on above amount:

To be depreciated.. .... $20,000

Remaining life .... 5 years

Depreciation expense in current year .... $ 4,000

To correct the error:

Operating income originally reported........ .... $160,000

Increase in repair expense............ .... (20,000)

Decrease in depreciation expense.. 4,000

Corrected operating income.......... .... **$144,000**

b. ***ROI for current year based on original data:***

ROI = Operating income / Average total assets

= $160,000 / (($940,000 + $1,020,000) / 2) = **16.3%**

ROI for current year based on corrected data:

Year-end assets originally reported.......... .... $1,020,000

Less net book value of mistakenly capitalized repair expense:

Cost $20,000

Less accumulated depreciation..... .... (4,000)   (16,000)

Corrected year-end assets $1,004,000

ROI = Operating income / Average total assets

= $144,000 / (($940,000 + $1,004,000) / 2) = **14.8%**

c. In subsequent years, depreciation expense will be too high, net income will be too low, and average assets will be too high. Thus, ROI will be too low.

P6-17. a. Estimated useful life .... 5 years

Cost of machine $44,000

Estimated salvage value................ .... (6,000)

Amount to be depreciated $38,000

1. Straight-line depreciation:

Annual depreciation expense = $38,000 / 5 = **$7,600 per year**

P6-17. a. 2. *Sum-of-the-years-digits depreciation:*
Sum of the digits for a 5-year life = (5 + 4 +3 +2 + 1) = 15 digits

Year	Depreciation Expense
1	5/15 * $38,000 = **$12,667**
2	4/15 * 38,000 = **10,133**
3	3/15 * 38,000 = **7,600**
4	2/15 * 38,000 = **5,067**
5	1/15 * 38,000 = **2,533**
Total	$38,000

3. *Double-declining-balance depreciation:*
Straight-line rate = 1 / 5 = 20%. Double-declining rate = 20% * 2 = **40%**

	Net Book Value	Depreciation	At End of Year Accumulated	Net Book
Year	at Beginning of Year	Expense	Depreciation	Value
1	$44,000	$44,000 * 40% = $17,600	$17,600	$26,400
2	26,400	26,400 * 40% = 10,560	28,160	15,840
3	15,840	15,840 * 40% = 6,336	34,496	9,504
4	9,504	9,504 * 40% = 3,801#	38,297	5,703#

\# This is the calculated amount, but the net book value cannot go below salvage
value, so depreciation expense in the fourth year is limited to $3,504, as follows:

4	9,504	3,504	38,000	6,000
5	6,000	0	38,000	6,000

4. *150% Declining-balance depreciation:*
Straight-line rate = 1 / 5 = 20%. 150% declining rate = 20% * 1.5 = **30%**

	Net Book Value	Depreciation	At End of Year Accumulated	Net Book
Year	at Beginning of Year	Expense	Depreciation	Value
1	$44,000	$44,000 * 30% = $13,200	$13,200	$30,800
2	30,800	30,800 * 30% = 9,240	22,440	21,560
3	21,560	21,560 * 30% = 6,468	28,908	15,092
4	15,092	15,092 * 30% = 4,528	33,436	10,564
5	10,564	10,564 * 30% = 3,169#	36,605	7,395#

P6-17. a. 4. *(continued)*

This is the calculated amount, but the net book value at the end of the asset's useful life should be equal to its estimated salvage value. Thus, Freedom Co. would have to record an additional $1,395 of depreciation expense in the fifth year ($7,395 net book value at the end of year five - $6,000 salvage value). Thus, total depreciation expense in the fifth year would be $4,564 ($3,169 computed amount + $1,395 required adjustment). An alternative approach would be to record $1,395 as depreciation expense in the sixth year of the asset's life (assuming that the machine is still being used).

b. One-half of the first year's depreciation expense should be recorded.

Straight-line = $7,600 * 6/12 = **$3,800**
Sum-of-the-year's-digits = $12,667 * 6/12 = **$6,334**
Double-declining-balance = $17,600 * 6/12 = **$8,800**
150% declining-balance = $13,200 * 6/12 = **$6,600**

c. At 12/31/02 (after 1½ years):

	Cost	*Accumulated Depreciation*	*Net Book Value*
Straight-line	$44,000	**$11,400**	**$32,600**
Sum-of-the-years-digits	44,000	**17,734#**	**26,266**
Double-declining-balance	44,000	**22,880#**	**21,120**
150% declining-balance	44,000	**17,820#**	**26,180**

Note: The accumulated depreciation is the first year's depreciation expense plus one-half of the second year's depreciation expense.

P6-19.

Estimated useful life..	4 years
Cost of machine	$120,000
Estimated salvage value...	(20,000)
Amount to be depreciated	$100,000

a.

Year	*Net Book Value at Beginning of Year*	*Net Book Value at End of Year*	*Depreciation Expense*	*Accumulated Depreciation*
2001	$120,000	$80,000	**$40,000**	$ 40,000
2002	80,000	50,000	**30,000**	70,000
2003	50,000	30,000	**20,000**	90,000
2004	30,000	20,000	**10,000**	100,000

P6-19. a. *(continued)*

The **sum-of-the-years'-digits method** is being used because the depreciation expense recorded each year is decreasing at a constant rate representing the 4/10, 3/10, 2/10, 1/10 pattern * $100,000.

b.

Year	Net Book Value at Beginning of Year	Net Book Value at End of Year	Depreciation Expense	Accumulated Depreciation
2001	$120,000	$98,000	**$22,000**	$ 22,000
2002	98,000	66,000	**32,000**	54,000
2003	66,000	38,000	**28,000**	82,000
2004	38,000	20,000	**18,000**	100,000

The **units of production method** is being used. At first glance, no clear pattern can be seen in the amount of depreciation expense recorded each year. However, based on the machine's productive capacity of 50,000 units and the actual production data provided for 2001-2004, the depreciation expense amounts shown above can be easily verified.

c.

Year	Net Book Value at Beginning of Year	Net Book Value at End of Year	Depreciation Expense	Accumulated Depreciation
2001	$120,000	$60,000	**$60,000**	$ 60,000
2002	60,000	30,000	**30,000**	90,000
2003	30,000	20,000	**10,000**	100,000
2004	20,000	20,000	**0**	100,000

The **double-declining balance (200%) method** is being used. Notice that the expense pattern is extremely accelerated in this case. Using the double-declining balance method for an asset with a 4-year useful life results in an annual depreciation rate of 50% (25% straight-line rate * 2) of the asset's net book value. In year 2003, the machine became fully depreciated after only $10,000 was recorded as depreciation expense, even though the calculated amount was higher (50% * $30,000 = $15,000).

d.

Year	Net Book Value at Beginning of Year	Net Book Value at End of Year	Depreciation Expense	Accumulated Depreciation
2001	$120,000	$95,000	**$25,000**	$ 25,000
2002	95,000	70,000	**25,000**	50,000
2003	70,000	45,000	**25,000**	75,000
2004	45,000	20,000	**25,000**	100,000

The **straight-line method** is being used because an equal amount of depreciation expense is recorded each year, which represents 1/4 * $100,000.

P6-21. a. Depreciation expense for 2002 is the *increase* in the amount of accumulated depreciation from the beginning balance sheet to the ending balance sheet, or $18,000 ($42,000 – $24,000).

    b. 1. The cost of the asset is the net book value plus the accumulated depreciation, or $28,000 + $42,000 = **$70,000.**

        2. It is difficult to determine which depreciation *method* is being used because the acquisition date of the asset is not known. However, the *amount* to be depreciated can be determined, as follows:

Estimated useful life	4 years
Cost of machine	$70,000
Estimated salvage value	(10,000)
Amount to be depreciated	$60,000

The straight-line method is not being used because the annual depreciation expense would be $15,000 ($60,000 / 4 years), and not $18,000 as determined in part *a*.

The **sum-of the-years'-digits method** is being used because the balance of the accumulated depreciation account has increased from $24,000 to $42,000, which is consistent with the depreciation pattern under this method. For an asset with a 4-year useful life, the depreciation pattern would be: 4/10, 3/10, 2/10, 1/10.

		At End of Year	
Year	*Depreciation Expense*	*Accumulated Depreciation*	*Net Book Value*
1	4/10 * $60,000 = **$24,000**	**$24,000**	**$46,000**
2	3/10 * 60,000 = **18,000**	42,000	28,000
3	2/10 * 60,000 = 12,000	54,000	16,000
4	1/10 * 60,000 = 6,000	60,000	10,000

        3. At December 31, 2002, the accumulated depreciation of $42,000 represents 2 years of depreciation expense, so the acquisition date of the machine must have been on or near **January 1, 2001.**

c.

Dr. Cash	$23,600
Dr. Accumulated depreciation	42,000
Dr. Loss on sale of machine	4,400
Cr. Machine	$70,000

    To record the sale of a machine at a loss.

P6-21. c. *(continued)*

Balance Sheet				Income Statement		
Assets	= Liabilities	+ Owners' Equity	← Net income	= Revenues	-	Expenses
Cash						Loss on Sale
+23,600						of Machine
Machine						−4,400
−70,000						
Accumulated	*(A decrease in a*					
Depreciation	*contra-asset account*					
+42,000	*increases assets).*					

P6-23. a. If *any* of the four criteria listed in the text for capitalizing a lease are met, the lease should be accounted for as a capital lease rather than an operating lease.

1. Maybe. The problem does not state that *ownership* of the computer system is transferred to Carey, Inc. during the term of the lease, but it does state that the system was *acquired*. Thus, its not clear whether title to the asset transferred.

2. Yes. The option to purchase the computer system for $1 at the end of four years is a "bargain purchase option."

3. Yes. The 75% test is met because the lease term of 4 years is 100% of the economic life of the computer system.

4. Yes. The 90% test is met because the present value of the lease payments is $10,197.95 which is 100% (rounded) of the $10,200 fair value of the asset.

b. Annual lease payments (paid at the end of each year)...... .... $ 3,500
Present value factor (Table 6-3, 4 periods, 14% discount rate)... .... * 2.9137
Present value of lease payments (amount to be capitalized)........ .... **$10,197.95**

Dr. Equipment.... .... $10,200
    Cr. Capital Lease Liability $10,200
    To record a capital lease transaction at the present value of future lease
    payments (amount rounded to the nearest $10).

P6-23. b. *(continued)*

Balance Sheet			Income Statement		
Assets =	**Liabilities** +	**Owners' Equity** ←	**Net income** =	**Revenues** -	**Expenses**
Equipment	Capital				
+ 10,200	Lease Liability				
	+ 10,200				

c. Annual lease payment .... $ 3,500
  Beginning balance, capital lease liability... .... $10,200
  Interest rate .... * 14%
  Interest expense (for first year of lease term) .... **(1,428)**
  Payment of principal (reduction of capital lease liability). **$2,072**

Dr. Interest Expense.................. .... $1,428
Dr. Capital Lease Liability.........   2,072
  Cr. Cash....... .... $3,500
  To record the first annual lease payment on a capital lease.

Balance Sheet			Income Statement		
Assets =	**Liabilities** +	**Owners' Equity** ←	**Net income** =	**Revenues** -	**Expenses**
Cash	Capital				Interest
– 3,500	Lease Liability				Expense
	– 2,072				– 1,428

d. In addition to the **$1,428 of Interest Expense** on the capital lease liability, **Depreciation Expense of $2,550** ($10,200 / 4 years) on the equipment should also be recognized in the income statement. Note that the amount of interest expense will *decrease* each year of the lease term because the capital lease liability is reduced each time an annual lease payment is made.

e. As discussed and illustrated in the text, the *economic effect* of a long-term capital lease is not any different than the purchase of an asset with borrowed funds. In substance, the f firm has acquired virtually all of the rights and benefits of ownership—so the accounting for a capital lease should be consistent with that of an asset purchase.

P6-25. a. The cost of the machine at the beginning of the lease is the present value of the lease payments discounted at the interest rate the lessor would charge. $900 per year is an annuity. The present value factor for an annuity of 10 periods, at a discount rate of 12% in Table 6-3 is 5.6502. Thus, the present value of the lease payments is:
  $900 * 5.6502 = **$5,085**

P6-25. b. The difference between the total amount paid and the present value of the lease payments is interest.

c. The cost to be reported in Renter's balance sheet is the present value of the lease payments, **$5,085.**

Accounting for and Presentation of Liabilities

E7-1. Discount basis means interest is paid in advance.

   a. Proceeds = Face amount of note − Interest
        = $300,000 − ($300,000 * 9% * 6/12)
        = $300,000 − $13,500 = **$286,500**

April 15, 2002

Dr. Cash.....	$286,500	
Dr. Discount on Notes Payable......	13,500	
Cr. Notes Payable..................		$300,000

To record the proceeds of a short-term note payable (discount basis).

Balance Sheet			Income Statement		
Assets =	**Liabilities** +	**Owners' Equity**	← **Net income** =	**Revenues** -	**Expenses**

Cash	Notes Payable	*(Note: The discount account is a contra liability,*
+ 286,500	+ 300,000	*so the initial carrying value of the note is equal*
	Discount on	*to the cash proceeds received--which is the*
	Notes Payable	*approach taken when interest is calculated*
	− 13,500	*on a straight basis.)*

   b. The note was dated April 15, 2002, so 2½ months have passed from the time the note was signed until the June 30, 2002 fiscal year-end. Interest = $300,000 * 9% * 2½/12 = **$5,625**

   c. Current liability = Face amount less discount balance.
        = $300,000 − ($13,500 − $5,625)
        = $300,000 − $7,875 = **$292,125**

E7-3. a. *3/31/02*

Dr. Payroll Tax Expense.............	$4,800	
Cr. Payroll Taxes Payable......		$4,800

To accrue payroll taxes for the year.

Balance Sheet			Income Statement		
Assets =	**Liabilities** +	**Owners' Equity**	← **Net income** =	**Revenues** -	**Expenses**
	Payroll Taxes				Payroll Tax
	Payable				Expense
	+ 4,800				− 4,800

E7-3. b. Failure to make the accrual resulted in an understatement of expense and an overstatement of net income. On the 3/31/02 balance sheet, current liabilities are understated and retained earnings is overstated.

c.

3/31/02	3/31/03

Paid taxes of prior year in April; debited expense for $4,800 this year.

Should have recognized $5,000 expense this year.

Effect on net income for year ended 3/31/03:
Expense is too high by amount applicable to prior year: $4,800
Expense is too low by accrual *not* made this year: $5,000
Net effect is that expense this year is $200 too low, and profits this year are $200 too high.

Effect on the 3/31/03 balance sheet:
Current liabilities are $5,000 understated, and retained earnings is $5,000 overstated.

E7-5. a. Warranty Expense = ($3,600,000 sales * 0.4% estimated warranty expense) = **$14,400**

b.

Estimated Warranty Liability, 1/1/02 balance	$35,200
Less: Actual warranty costs during 2002	(15,600)
Add: Warranty Expense accrued during 2002	14,400
Estimated Warranty Liability, 12/31/02 balance	$34,000

E7-7. a. Keg deposits are a current liability on the balance sheet because they are amounts that are likely to be paid within a year.

b. Dr. Keg Deposits. $50

     Cr. Cash......... .... $50

      To record the refund of keg deposits.

Balance Sheet			Income Statement		
Assets =	**Liabilities** +	**Owners' Equity** ←	**Net income** =	**Revenues** -	**Expenses**
Cash	Keg Deposits				
– 50	– 50				

E7-7. c. The Keg Deposits liability for the 200 kegs (200 * $50 = $10,000) should be eliminated with a debit; an income statement account (such as Keg Deposits Revenue) should be credited.

Dr. Keg Deposits	$10,000	
Cr. Keg Deposits Revenue		$10,000

To eliminate the liability for   unreturned kegs.

Balance Sheet	Income Statement
Assets = Liabilities + Owners' Equity ←	**Net income = Revenues - Expenses**
To eliminate the liability for unreturned kegs:	
Keg Deposits	Keg Deposits
– 10,000	Revenue
	+10,000

d. The cost of kegs purchased would be capitalized in a long-lived asset account, and then be depreciated over the kegs' estimated useful life. The net book value of kegs removed from service or lost (as in part *c*) would be removed from the asset and recorded as an expense (or a loss).

Dr. Keg Expense (or Loss on Unreturned Kegs)	$ xxx	
Dr. Accumulated Depreciation	xxx	
Cr. Kegs (or other appropriate asset account)...........		$ xxx

To record a loss for the net book value of unreturned kegs.

Balance Sheet	Income Statement
Assets = Liabilities + Owners' Equity ←	**Net income = Revenues - Expenses**
To record a loss for the net book value of unreturned kegs:	
– Kegs	– Keg Expense
+ Accumulated	*(or Unreturned*
Depreciation	*Kegs Loss)*

E7-9. a. The market interest rate is lower than the stated interest rate, so the bonds will sell for more than their face amount. The lower the discount rate (i.e., market interest rate), the higher the *present value* of cash flows associated with the bond (for interest payments and principal) becomes.

b. Dr. Cash	$1,080,000	
Cr. Bonds Payable..............		$1,000,000
Cr. Premium on Bonds Payable		80,000

To record the issuance of bonds payable at a premium.

E7-9. b. *(continued)*

	Balance Sheet			**Income Statement**		
Assets	**=**	**Liabilities**	**+ Owners' Equity** ←	**Net income**	**= Revenues**	**- Expenses**
Cash		Bonds Payable				
+1,080,000		+1,000,000				
		Premium on				
		Bonds Payable				
		+80,000				

c.

4/1/02	6 months	9/30/02
Bonds issued.		End of fiscal year.

Accrued interest payable ($1,000,000 * 11% * 6/12)....... .... $55,000
Premium amortization ($80,000 / 20 years * 6/12)........... ....   (2,000)
Interest expense for 6 months....... ....   **$53,000**

Dr. Interest Expense $53,000
Dr. Premium on Bonds Payable..   2,000
    Cr. Interest Payable............... .... $55,000
      To record the accrual of interest and premium amortization for 6 months.

E7-11. The semiannual interest on the bonds = 10% stated rate * $5,000 face amount
* 6/12 = **$250**

The remaining term of the bonds is 12 years, or **24 semiannual periods.**

The semiannual market interest rate is = 8% * 6/12 = **4%**

The present value of an interest annuity of $250 for 24 periods at 4% =
$250 * 15.2470 = **$3,811.75**

The present value of the maturity value of $5,000 in 24 periods at 4% =
$5,000 * 0.3901 = **$1,950.50**

The market value of the bonds = PV of interest + PV of maturity value =
$3,811.75 + $1,950.50 = **$5,762.25**

E7-13. a. Annual interest payment = $40 million * 11% = **$4,400,000**

    b. The bonds were issued at a discount because market interest rates were more than the stated rate when the bonds were issued. The higher the discount rate (i.e., the market interest rate), the lower the *present value* of cash flows for interest payments and principal (i.e., the lower the bond's selling price).

    c. Interest expense will be more than the interest paid because the amortization of bond discount will increase interest expense.

E7-15. The principal risk associated with financial leverage is that a decrease in the entity's operating income could result in a decrease in cash flows and an inability to make interest and required principal payments on the debt. A second risk is that as the amount of debt increases, lenders require a higher interest rate to compensate for the additional risk they are taking.

E7-17. The amount of deferred income taxes has risen steadily because the excess of accelerated tax depreciation over straight-line book depreciation on recent asset additions exceeds the excess of book depreciation over tax depreciation for older asset additions. This occurs because as the company grows over time, asset additions increase in amount, and over time the cost of replacement assets rises because of inflation.

E7-19. *Transaction/ Adjustment*	*Current Assets*	*Current Liabilities*	*Long-Term Debt*	*Net Income*
a.		+867		-867
b.		+170		-170
c.		+1,700		-1,700
d.			+50	-50
e.	-1,240	- 1,240		
f.		+1,500		-1,500

E7-19. *Journal entries:*

a. Dr. Wages Expense .... $ 867
     Cr. Wages Payable .... $ 867

b. Dr. Interest Expense............. 170
     Cr. Interest Payable........... 170

c. Dr. Interest Expense ($240,000 * 8.5% * 1/12) 1,700
     Cr.   Interest Payable........... 1,700

d. Dr. Interest Expense 50
     Cr. Discount on Bonds Payable 50

e. Dr. Estimated Warranty Liability 1,240
     Cr. Cash...... 410
     Cr. Parts Inventory............ 830

f. Dr. Sales 1,500
     Cr. Unearned Revenues....... 1,500

E7-21.

Transaction/ Adjustment	Current Assets	Noncurrent Assets	Current Liabilities	Noncurrent Liabilities	Owners' Equity	Net Income
a.			Income Taxes Payable + 500	Deferred Income Taxes + 200		Income Tax Expense – 700
b.	Cash + 4,950			Bonds Payable + 5,000 Discount on Bonds Payable – 50		
c.	Cash – 3,000	Land + 3,000				
d.	Inventory – 64		Estimated Warranty Liability – 64			

E7-21. *Transaction/ Adjustment*	*Current Assets*	*Noncurrent Assets*	*Current Liabilities*	*Noncurrent Liabilities*	*Owners' Equity*	*Net Income*
e.	Cash + 19,400		Notes Payable + 20,000 Discount on Notes Payable – 600			
f.			Current Maturities of Long-Term Debt + 35,000	Serial Bonds Payable – 35,000		

Journal entries:

a. Dr. Income Tax Expense .... $ 700
    Cr. Income Taxes Payable .... $ 500
    Cr. Deferred Income Taxes 200

b. Dr. Cash.. 4,950
    Dr. Discount on Bonds Payable 50
    Cr. Bonds Payable................ 5,000

c. Dr. Land.. 3,000
    Cr. Cash....... 3,000

d. Dr. Estimated Warranty Liability 64
    Cr. Inventory. 64

e. Dr. Cash ($20,000 – ($20,000 * 12% * 3/12)).. 19,400
    Dr. Discount on Notes Payable ($20,000 * 12% * 3/12) 600
    Cr. Notes Payable................ 20,000

f. Dr. Serial Bonds Payable............ 35,000
    Cr. Current Maturities of Long-Term Debt.. 35,000

P7-23. a. *September 1, 2001*
    Dr. Cash. $4,200
    Cr. Unearned Rent Revenue $4,200
      To record the receipt a six-month advance rent payment.

P7-23. a. *(continued)*

Each month-end:
Dr.   Unearned Rent Revenue........ .... $700
    Cr.   Rent Revenue.................. .... $700
<small>To record a reduction in the liability account for rent earned each month.</small>

Balance Sheet			Income Statement		
Assets =	**Liabilities** +	**Owners' Equity**	← **Net income** =	**Revenues** -	**Expenses**
Cash	Unearned				
+ 4,200	Rent Revenue				
	+ 4,200				
	Unearned			Rent	
	Rent Revenue			Revenue	
	− 700			+ 700	

b. At December 31, 2001, 4 months of rent has been earned, and 2 months remains to be earned. So 2/6 of the original premium of $4,200, or $1,400 is unearned rent and will be shown on the December 31 balance sheet as a current liability.

c. At a rate of $700 per month, the receipt of an 18-month rent prepayment would have been for $12,600. The unearned amount at December 31, 2001, is $9,800 ($700 per month for the next 14 months). Only $8,400 ($700 * 12 months) of this amount is a current liability, because of the one-year time frame for current liabilities. Thus, $1,400 ($700 * 2 months) of the unearned amount is technically a noncurrent liability.

P7-25.   a. Gross Pay – Total Deductions = Net Pay
       Gross Pay = (Net Pay + Total Deductions)
            = ($58,360 + $21,640) = **$80,000**

       FICA Tax Withholdings = (Total Deductions – all other deductions)
                = ($21,640 – $13,760 – $1,120 – $640) = **$6,120**

       FICA Tax Withholdings / Gross Pay = withholding percentage
              $6,120 / $80,000 = **7.65%**

P7-25. b. Dr. Wages Expense $80,000

                Cr. Wages Payable (or Accrued Payroll)..... .... $58,360

                Cr. FICA Taxes Withheld.... 6,120

                Cr. Income Taxes Withheld. 13,760

                Cr. Medical Insurance Contributions 1,120

                Cr. Union Dues 640

                To record accrued payroll.

Balance Sheet			Income Statement		
Assets =	**Liabilities** +	**Owners' Equity**	← **Net income** =	**Revenues** -	**Expenses**
	Wages Payable				Wages
	+ 58,360				Expense
	Withholding Liabilities (as described above)				−80,000
	+ 6,120 + 13,760 + 1,120 + 640				

P7-27. a. Because the exchange ratio is five shares of common stock to one bond, bondholders would be interested in converting the bonds to common stock if the market price per share of common stock was at least 20% (or more) of the market price per bond. For example, when the bonds were issued on January 1, 1993 at their $1,000 face amount, the market rate of interest and the stated rate were both 12%, and the market price per bond was $1,000. At that time, bondholders would not have been willing to convert their bonds unless the common stock was trading at price of $200 per share or more.

    b. ***Solution approach:*** Upon exercise of the conversion feature, the bonds have been retired and thus the Bonds Payable account must be reduced by the carrying value of $1,000 per bond retired (there was no discount or premium). Common stock has been issued for $215 per share and should be recorded in the usual way. The difference is a loss on the early retirement of bonds of $75 per bond retired (or $15 per share of common stock issued) because the company gave more in exchange for the bonds ($215 per share * 5 shares equals $1,075) than the carrying value of the bonds ($1,000 per bond).

      Dr. Bonds Payable (400 bonds * $1,000 per bond)....... .... $400,000

      Dr. Loss on Early Retirement of Bonds # 30,000

         Cr. Common Stock (400 bonds * 5 shares * $10 par)............ $ 20,000

         Cr. Additional Paid-In Capital (400 * 5 * $205 per share).. 410,000

         To record the conversion of bonds to common stock at a loss.

       # For financial reporting purposes, gains and losses on the early retirement of debt are reported as "extraordinary items" on the income statement, and are shown net of their tax effects. The accounting for extraordinary items is discussed in Chapter 9.

P7-27. b. *(continued)*

Balance Sheet				Income Statement		
Assets	=	Liabilities	+ Owners' Equity	← Net income =	Revenues -	Expenses
		Bonds	Common Stock			Loss on
		Payable	+ 20,000			Early
		– 400,000	Additional Paid-In			Retirement
			Capital			of Bonds
			+ 410,000			– 30,000

P7-29. a. The semiannual interest payments on the bonds =
14% stated rate * $3,000,000 face amount * 6/12 = **$210,000**

The term of the bonds is 10 years, or **20 semiannual periods.**
The semiannual market interest rate is = 12% * 6/12 = **6%**

The present value of an annuity of $210,000 for 20 periods at 6% =
$210,000 * 11.4699 = **$2,408,679**

The present value of the maturity value of $3,000,000 in 20 periods at 6% =
$3,000,000 * 0.3118 = **$935,400**

The proceeds (issue price) of the bonds = PV of interest + PV of maturity value =
$2,408,679 + $935,400 = **$3,344,079**

b. The semiannual discount amortization, straight-line basis = $50,000 / 20 periods = **$2,500**

Dr. Interest Expense................... .... $212,500
    Cr. Cash........ .... $210,000
    Cr. Discount on Bonds Payable 2,500
To record the semiannual cash payment and amortization of discount.

Balance Sheet				Income Statement		
Assets	=	Liabilities	+ Owners' Equity	← Net income =	Revenues -	Expenses
Cash		Discount on				Interest
– 210,000		Bonds Payable				Expense
		+ 2,500				– 212,500

    146

P7-29. c. Discount on bonds payable is amortized with a credit, and thus increases interest expense. Under the straight-line basis, the amount of discount amortization is the same each period. Under the compound (or *effective*) interest method, the amount of discount amortization increases each period. Thus, interest expense under the compound method will be lower in the early years of the bond's life, and higher in the later years, as compared to interest expense under the straight-line method of amortization.

Rationale of compound interest method: <u>*Interest expense*</u> under the compound interest method is calculated by multiplying the carrying value of the bond (face amount minus the unamortized discount) by the market rate of interest. This amount is then compared to the <u>*cash payment*</u> required (the face amount multiplied by the stated rate). Any difference between interest expense and the required cash payment represents the amortization of discount for the period. Because the carrying value of the bond *increases* over the life of the bond as discount is amortized, the *amount* of discount amortization also increases each period, causing interest expense to be higher each period. Thus, as compared to the straight-line basis, interest expense under the compound method will be lower in the first year.

Accounting for and Presentation of Owners' Equity

E8-1.

	A	=	**L**	+	**OE**		
					PIC	+	**RE**
Beginning..........	$ (4)		$ (3)		(1)		(2) $520,000 OE
Changes	+260,000		+21,000		+40,000		+ (7) Net income
							−55,000 Dividends
Ending	(5)	=	$234,000	+	$175,000	+	(6)

Steps:
1. $175,000 − $40,000 = $135,000
2. $520,000 − $135,000 = $385,000
3. $234,000 − $21,000 = $213,000
4. $213,000 + $520,000 = $733,000
5. $733,000 + $260,000 = $993,000
6. $993,000 − $234,000 − $175,000 = $584,000
7. $385,000 + Net income − $55,000 = $584,000
    Net income = **$254,000**

Short-cut approach:
$260,000 = + $21,000 + $40,000
       + Net income − $55,000

     Net income = **$254,000**

E8-3.
Retained earnings, December 31, 2001	$346,400
Add: Net income for the year	56,900
Less: Dividends for the year	(32,500)
Retained earnings, December 31, 2002	**$370,800**

E8-5. a. Balance sheet amount equals number of shares issued * par value.
    1,400,000 shares * $5 = **$7,000,000**

  b. Cash dividends are paid on shares outstanding.
    1,250,000 shares * $0.15 = **$187,500**

  c. Treasury stock accounts for the difference between shares issued and shares outstanding.

E8-7.
a. Number of shares issued	161,522
Less: Number of shares in treasury	(43,373)
Number of shares outstanding	118,149
Dividend requirement per share	* $3.75
Total annual dividends required to be paid..	**$443,058.75**

E8-7. b. Dividend per share (6% * $40 par value) $2.40
      Number of shares outstanding   73,621
      Total annual dividends required to be paid.. ....   **$176,690.40**

     c. Dividend per share (11.4% * $100 stated value) $11.40
      Number of shares outstanding   37,600
      Total annual dividends required to be paid.. ....   **$428,640**

E8-9. Preferred dividends for 2000, 2001, and 2002 would have to be paid before a dividend on the common stock could be paid. Annual dividend = $6.50 * 22,000 shares = $143,000 Dividends for 3 years = 3 * $143,000 = **$429,000**

E8-11. a. February 21 is the declaration date. Because this is a regular dividend of the same amount as prior dividends, the stock price would not be significantly affected.

     b. March 12 is the ex-dividend date. On this date the market price of the stock is likely to fall by the amount of the dividend because purchasers will not receive the dividend.

     c. March 15 is the record date. The market price of the stock should not be affected because for a publicly traded stock it is the ex-dividend date that affects who receives the dividend.

     d. March 30 is the payment date. The market price of the stock should not be affected because the corporation is merely paying a liability (dividends payable).

E8-13. To declare a dividend, the firm must have retained earnings and enough cash to pay the dividend. Of course the board of directors must approve a dividend.

E8-15. If the company can reinvest its retained earnings at a higher ROI than I could earn on the money paid to me in dividends, I would prefer that the company *not* pay a cash dividend (Intel is a perfect example of this). If I needed current income from my investment, I would want cash dividends. As a common stock investor, I don't really care whether or not the company issues a stock dividend, because a stock dividend doesn't change my equity in the company, the total market value of my investment, or the company's ability to earn a return on my investment.

E8-17. a. A 2-for-1 split means that for every share now owned, the stockholder will own 2 shares. Thus, I will own 200 shares.

b. Because there are now twice as many shares of stock outstanding, and the financial condition of the company hasn't changed, the market price per share should be half of what it was, or $20 per share. The total market value of my investment will not have changed.

c. The par value per share is also likely to be split in half (i.e., from $10 to $5), but this does not happen automatically—any changes in par value per share require action by the board of directors.

P8-19. a. 1. *January 1, 2001:*

Dr. Cash ((150,000 @ $19) + (60,000 @ $122))................. .... $10,170,000
    Cr. Common Stock (150,000 shares @ $19 per share)...... .... $2,850,000
    Cr. Preferred Stock (60,000 shares @ $100 per share)......   6,000,000
    Cr. Additional Paid-In Capital--Preferred (60,000 @ $22)   1,320,000
    To record stock issuances.

2. *December 28, 2002:*

Dr. Retained Earnings $1,800,000
    Cr. Dividends Payable $1,800,000
    To record the declaration of dividends.

3. *February 12, 2003:*

Dr. Dividends Payable................. .... $1,800,000
    Cr. Cash.......... .... $1,800,000
    To record the payment of dividends.

Balance Sheet			Income Statement	
Assets =	Liabilities +	Owners' Equity	← Net income =	Revenues - Expense

1. *To record stock issuances:*

Cash	Common Stock			
+ 10,170,000	+ 2,850,000			
	Preferred Stock			
	+ 6,000,000			
	Additional			
	Paid-In Capital			
	+ 1,320,000			

P8-19. a. *(continued)*

Balance Sheet				Income Statement		
Assets	=	**Liabilities**	+ **Owners' Equity**	← **Net income**	= **Revenues**	- **Expense**

    2. *To record the declaration of dividends:*

	Dividends	Retained
	Payable	Earnings
	+ 1,800,000	– 1,800,000

    3. *To record the payment of dividends:*

Cash	Dividends
– 1,800,000	Payable
	– 1,800,000

b. Preferred shareholders are entitled to one year of dividends in arrears (for 2001), as well as their current year preference (for 2002). 60,000 shares * $100 par per share * 9.5% = $570,000 per year * 2 years = **$1,140,000**

P8-21. a. *May 4, 2002:*

Dr. Treasury Stock..........................	$14,600	
Cr. Cash........		$14,600
To record the purchase of 800 shares of treasury stock @ $18.25 per share.		

June 15, 2002:

Dr. Retained Earnings (36,200 – 800 = 35,400 shares * $0.35).	12,390	
Cr. Cash........		12,390
To record the declaration and payment of a cash dividend.		

September 11, 2002:

Dr. Cash (600 shares @ $19.50)........	11,700	
Cr. Treasury Stock (600 shares @ $18.25)........		10,950
Cr. Additional Paid-In Capital (600 shares @ $1.25).....		750
To record the sale of 600 shares of treasury stock @ $19.50 per share.		

Balance Sheet			Income Statement		
Assets	=	**Liabilities** + **Owners' Equity**	← **Net income**	= **Revenues**	- **Expenses**

To record the purchase of 800 shares of treasury stock @ $18.25 per share:

Cash	Treasury Stock
– 14,600	– 14,600

P8-21. a. *(continued)*

Balance Sheet			Income Statement		
Assets =	**Liabilities** +	**Owners' Equity**	← **Net income** =	**Revenues** -	**Expenses**

To record the declaration and payment of a cash dividend:

Cash
– 12,390

Retained
Earnings
– 12,390

To record the sale of 600 shares of treasury stock @ $19.50 per share.

Cash
+ 11,700

Treasury Stock
+ 10,950
Additional
Paid-in Capital
+ 750

P8-23.

Transaction	Cash	Other Assets	Liabilities	Paid-in Capital	Retained Earnings	Treasury Stock *	Net Income
a.	+205,000			+205,000			
b.			+18,450		–18,450		
c.	–35,100					+35,100	
d.		+113,000		+113,000			
e.	+17,400			+1,200		–16,200	
f.	No entry is required for a stock split.						

* Note that an increase in treasury stock (for a purchase transaction such as item c) decreases total owners' equity, and a decrease in treasury stock (for a sale transaction such as item e) increases total owners' equity. The effects shown are with respect to the Treasury Stock account, which is a contra owners' equity account.

Journal entries:

a. Dr. Cash ($50 par * 4,100 shares)....... .... $205,000
   Cr. Preferred Stock $205,000

b. Dr. Retained Earnings ($50 par * 9% * 4,100 shares) 18,450
   Cr. Dividends Payable 18,450

c. Dr. Treasury Stock ($54 per share * 650 shares) 35,100
   Cr. Cash....... 35,100

d. Dr. Land (market value) 113,000
   Cr. Common Stock ($1 par * 2,000 shares) 2,000
   Cr. Additional Paid-In Capital (excess over par).......... 111,000

P8-23. e. Dr.   Cash ($58 per share * 300 shares) $17,400
  Cr.   Treasury Stock ($54 per share * 300 shares). $16,200
  Cr.   Additional Paid-In Capital ($4 excess * 300 shares)   1,200
  f.   No entry is required for a stock split.

P8-25.

Transaction	Cash	Other Assets	Liabilities	Paid-in Capital	Retained Earnings	Treasury Stock *	Net Income
a.	+ 90,000			+ 90,000			
b.		+ 40,000		+ 40,000			
c.	− 3,200				− 3,200		
d.	− 4,750					+ 4,750	
e.			+ 6,713		− 6,713		
f.	+ 2,600			+ 130		− 2,470	
g.				+ 28,350	− 28,350		

h.   No entry is required for a stock split.

* Note that an increase in treasury stock (for a purchase transaction such as item d) decreases total owners' equity, and a decrease in treasury stock (for a sale transaction such as item f) increases total owners' equity. The effects shown are with respect to the Treasury Stock account, which is a contra owners' equity account.

Journal entries:

a. Dr. Cash... .... $90,000
  Cr.   Common Stock ($1 per share * 5,000 shares)... .... $ 5,000
  Cr.   Additional Paid-In Capital ($17 per share * 5,000 shares)   85,000

b. Dr. Land and Building 40,000
  Cr.   Preferred Stock ($40 per share * 1,000 shares)   40,000

c. Dr. Retained Earnings ($40 per share * 8% * 1,000 shares) 3,200
  Cr.   Cash..........   3,200

d. Dr. Treasury Stock ($4,750 / 250 shares = $19 per share).......... 4,750
  Cr.   Cash........   4,750

e. Dr. Retained Earnings (40,000 + 5,000 − 250 = 44,750 shares) 6,713
  Cr.   Dividends Payable ($0.15 per share * 44,750 shares outstanding)   6,713

f. Dr. Cash ($20 per share * 130 shares). 2,600
  Cr.   Treasury Stock ($19 per share * 130 shares)   2,470
  Cr.   Additional Paid-In Capital ($1 per share * 130 shares)   130

P8-25. g. Dr. Retained Earnings (45,000 shares *issued* * 3% = 1,350)... .... $28,350

Cr. Common Stock ($1 per share * 1,350 dividend shares) . ... $ 1,350
Cr. Additional Paid-In Capital ($20 per share * 1,350 per share)...   27,000

P8-27. a. Annual dividend per share (12% * $60)..... .... $ 7.20
Number of shares outstanding   1,500
Annual dividend requirement........ ....   **$10,800**

b. Balance sheet amount = ($60 par value * 1,500 shares issued) = **$90,000**

c. Number shares issued = ($240,000 balance sheet amount / $8 par value) = **30,000**
Number shares outstanding = (30,000 shares issued – 2,000 treasury shares) = **28,000**

d.

	Common Stock	*Additional Paid-in Capital*
November 30, 2002	$240,000	$540,000
January 1, 2002......	(210,000)	(468,750)
Increase......	**$ 30,000**	**$ 71,250**

Number of shares sold = ($30,000 increase in common stock / $8 par value) = **3,750**

Selling price per share = (($30,000 increase in common stock + $71,250 increase in additional paid-in capital) / 3,750 shares sold) = **$27 per share.**

e. Treasury stock was resold at a price greater than its cost.

f. Retained earnings, January 1, 2002 .... $90,300
Add: Net income....   24,000
Less: Preferred stock dividends *(see answer to part a)*...... ....   (10,800)
Less: Common stock dividends ....   ?
Retained earnings, December 31, 2002..... ....   **$97,000**

Solving for the unknown amount, common stock dividends = **$6,500**

The Income Statement and the Statement of Cash Flows

E9-1.

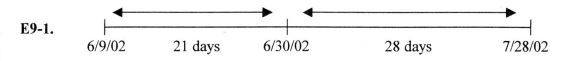

| 6/9/02 | 21 days | 6/30/02 | 28 days | 7/28/02 |

a. For the year end June 30, 2002, recognize 21/49 of summer school tuition, because that proportion of the summer session occurs within the first fiscal year. Summer session expenses will be accrued or deferred (i.e., recognized as incurred), so an appropriate matching of revenue and expense will occur in each fiscal year.

Amount of revenue for the year ended June 30, 2002 = (21/49 * $112,000) = **$48,000**

b. No. Revenues and expenses would still be allocated to each fiscal year to achieve the most appropriate matching (based on when revenues are *earned* and when expenses are *incurred*). Since revenues are earned as services are provided, the critical event is the offering of classes rather than the university's tuition refund policy. Thus, the amounts calculated in part *a* would still result in the most meaningful financial statements for each fiscal year.

E9-3. *Solution approach:* Use the cost of goods sold model with hypothetical data that are the same except for the item in error:

	"Error"	*"Correct"*
Beginning inventory	$100,000	$100,000
Add: Purchases	300,000	300,000
Goods available for sale	$400,000	$400,000
Less: Ending inventory	(125,000)	(75,000)
Cost of goods sold	$275,000	$325,000

The overstatement of ending inventory causes cost of good sold to be too low, so **gross profit and operating income are too high, or overstated, by $50,000.**

	(in millions)		
E9-5. a.	*1999*	*1998*	*1997*
Net revenues	$29,389	$26,273	$25,070
Cost of sales	(11,836)	(12,088)	(9,945)
Gross profit	$17,553	$14,185	$15,125
Gross profit ratio	59.7%	54.0%	60.3%

E9-5. b. Using the gross profit ratio for 1999 of 59.7%:

Net sales ($ millions).............	$10,600
Cost of goods sold (40.3%).......	(4,272)
Gross profit (59.7%)	$ 6,238

Alternative calculation: Some students may calculate a weighted average gross profit ratio for the three-year period from 1997-1999, as follows:

Total gross profit ($17,553 + $14,185 + $15,125).......	$46,863
/ Total net revenues ($29,389 + $26,273 + $25,070)	$80,732
Weighted average gross profit ratio.......	58.0%

Net sales ($ millions)...............	$10,600
Cost of goods sold (42.0%).....	(4,452)
Gross profit (58.0%)	$ 6,148

E9-7. I would prefer to have operating income data, because this describes how well management has done operating the business. Net income is important, but includes non-recurring items such as discontinued operations and extraordinary items. Thus, trends in operating income data are more likely to reflect the firm's ability to generate future earnings than are trends in net income data.

E9-9.

Net income..	$473,400
Less: Dividends required on preferred stock (38,000 shares * $4.50 per share)..	(171,000)
Net income available for common stockholders	$302,400
/ Number of common share outstanding........	105,000
= Earnings per share—basic	$2.88

E9-11. a. ($760,000 sales on account + $24,000 decrease in accounts receivable) = **$784,000** source of cash. Since accounts receivable decreased during the year, more accounts were collected in cash than were created by credit sales.

Accounts Receivable

Beginning balance	$???	Cash collections	
Sales on account	$760,000	from customers	**$784,000**
Ending balance	$??? - 24,000		

E9-11. b. ($148,000 income tax expense + $34,000 decrease in income taxes payable) = **$182,000** use of cash. Tax payments exceeded the current year's income tax expense because the payable account decreased.

Income Taxes Payable

		Beginning balance	$	???
Cash payments for taxes	$182,000	Income tax expense		148,000
		Ending balance	$???	-32,000

c. ($408,000 cost of goods sold + $14,000 increase in inventory − $19,000 increase in accounts payable) = **$403,000** use of cash. Cost of goods sold reflects inventory uses. Inventory purchases were greater than inventory uses because inventory increased during the year, but part of the inventory purchases were not paid for in cash because accounts payable also increased during the year.

Inventory

Beginning balance	$	???		
Inventory purchases		422,000	Cost of goods sold	$408,000
Ending balance	$??? + $14,000			

Accounts Payable

Beginning balance	$	???	
Cash paid to suppliers	**403,000**	Inventory purchases	$422,000
		Ending balance	$??? + $19,000

d. ($240,000 increase in net book value + $190,000 depreciation expense) = **$430,000** use of cash. Since depreciation is an expense that does not affect cash, the amount of cash paid to purchase new buildings exceeded the increase in net book value. *(Note: In some years, a firm may spend an enormous amount of cash to acquire new buildings and equipment, yet still report a decrease in net book value.)*

Buildings, net of Accumulated Depreciation

Beginning balance	$	???	
Purchase of buildings	**$430,000**	Depreciation expense	$190,000
Ending balance	$??? + $240,000		

E9-13. a. Intel uses the multiple-step format, but does not report gross profit separately. The multiple-step format seems easier to read and interpret because it provides intermediate captions and subtotals that are useful to investors.

   b. The EPS disclosures (basic and diluted) are important measures to investors because they express accrual accounting income on a per share basis. For Intel, these disclosures are straight-forward. As discussed in the text, however, additional disclosure about the significant elements of EPS is appropriate for any years during which a firm reports any of the "unusual" income statement items (i.e., the "net of tax" items—discontinued operations, extraordinary items, and/or cumulative effect of accounting changes). Knowledge about the impact of non-recurring items provides investors with a better basis for anticipating what may happen to EPS in the future.

E9-15. a.-d. Answers vary depending upon the company being analyzed.

P9-17. a.

Net sales ..	$644,000
Cost of goods sold	(368,000)
Gross profit	$276,000
General and administrative expenses	(143,000)
Advertising expense	(45,000)
Other selling expenses	(13,000)
Operating income.	**$ 75,000**

   b. *Note:* Since Manahan Co. did not report any interest expense, or other income or expense, the operating income amount calculated in part *a* also represents the firm's "Income before taxes."

Income before taxes (operating income) ..	$ 75,000
Income tax expense	(26,000)
Earnings before extraordinary item	$ 49,000
Extraordinary loss from flood, net of taxes of $35,000....	(105,000)
Net loss....	**$ (56,000)**

P9-19. ***Solution approach:*** Calculate ending inventory in the cost of goods sold model for the high (33%) and low (30%) gross profit ratios, and select the ratio that gives the highest ending inventory.

P9-19. *(continued)*

		Gross Profit Ratio		
Calculation:	*33%*		*30%*	*Sequence*
Sales		$142,680	$142,680	Given
Cost of goods sold:				
Beginning inventory	$ 63,590		$ 63,590	Given
Add: Purchases	118,652		118,652	Given
Goods available for sale..........	$182,242		$182,242	
Less: Ending inventory...........	**(86,646)**		(82,366)	3rd
Cost of goods sold		$(95,596)	$(99,876)	2nd
Gross profit....		**$ 47,084**	$ 42,804	1st *

* Gross profit percentage multiplied by sales.

Franklin Co.'s management would argue for using a 33% gross profit ratio for 2002 to the date of the tornado, because the higher the gross profit ratio, the higher the estimated ending inventory lost in the storm, and the greater the insurance claim.

P9-21. a. ***Cash flows from operating activities:***   *($000 omitted)*

Net income	$420
Add (deduct) items not affecting cash:	
Depreciation and amortization expense.....	320
Accounts receivable decrease	45
Inventory increase	(20)
Accounts payable decrease	(10)
Income tax payable increase	35
Net cash provided by operating activities..	**$790**

b. Net income is based on accrual accounting, and revenues may be *earned* before or after cash is received. Likewise, expenses may be *incurred* before or after cash payments are made. Thus, net income and cash flows provided by operations may differ because of the *timing* of cash receipts and payments. In addition to the timing issue, other adjustments to net income may be necessary to add back non-cash expenses (such as depreciation and amortization), or to remove the effects of non-operating transactions (such as the gains and losses from the sale of long-term assets). To adjust net income for timing differences, changes during the year in non-cash working capital items (i.e., current assets other than cash, and current liabilities) must be considered. If a current asset account increases or if a current liability account decreases during the year, the cash account balance is assumed to have decreased. If a current asset account decreases or if a current liability account increases, the cash balance is assumed to have increased. *(Note: Review the Business in Practice—Understanding Cash Flow Relationships— Indirect Method if you are having difficulty understanding these adjustments.)*

P9-23. *Solution approach:* Prepare a statement of cash flows–direct method *(see Exhibit 9-9).*

a. **Cash flows from operating activities:** *(in millions)*

Cash collected from customers …	$1,350
Interest and taxes paid	(90)
Cash paid to suppliers and employees	(810)
Net cash provided by operating activities	$ 450

b. **Cash flows from investing activities:**

Purchase of land and buildings…	$(170)
Proceeds from the sale of equipment	40
Net cash used for investing activities	$(130)

c. **Cash flows from financing activities:**

Payment of long-term debt	$ (220)
Issuance of preferred stock	300
Cash dividends declared and paid	(340)
Net cash used for financing activities	$(260)
d. Net increase in cash for the year	$ 60

P9-25. a.

HOEMAN, INC.
Balance Sheets
December 31, 2002, and 2001

Assets

Current assets:		2002	2001
Cash		$ 52,000	$ 46,000
Accounts receivable	(1)	124,000	134,000
Inventory ..		156,000	176,000
Total current assets	(2)	$332,000	$ 356,000
Land	(3)	140,000	140,000
Buildings…	(4)	415,000	290,000
Less: Accumulated depreciation …		(120,000)	(105,000)
Total land & buildings	(5)	$435,000	$ 325,000
Total assets	(6)	$767,000	$ 681,000

Liabilities

Current liabilities:			
Note payable		$ 155,000	$ 124,000
Accounts payable ..	(7)	167,000	197,000
Total current liabilities		$ 322,000	$ 321,000
⁻ Long-term debt	(11)	$ 192,000	$ 139,000

P9-25. a. *(continued)*

Owners' Equity

Common stock......		$ 50,000	$ 45,000
Retained earnings..	(9)	203,000	176,000
Total owners' equity.................	(10)	$ 253,000	$ 221,000
Total liabilities and owners' equity	(8)	$ 767,000	$ 681,000

Calculations:

1. $134,000 – $10,000 = $124,000
2. $52,000 + $124,000 + $156,000 = $332,000
3. Land is carried at historical cost = $140,000
4. $290,000 + $125,000 = $415,000
5. $140,000 + $415,000 – $120,000 = $435,000
6. $332,000 + $435,000 = $767,000
7. $322,000 – $155,000 = $167,000
8. Same as total assets = $767,000
9. $176,000 + $94,000 – $67,000 = $203,000
10. $50,000 + $203,000 = $253,000
11. $767,000 – $253,000 – $322,000 = $192,000

b.

HOEMAN, INC.
Statement of Cash Flows
For the Year Ended December 31, 2002

Cash flows from operating activities:

Net income	$ 94,000
Add (deduct) items not affecting cash:	
Depreciation expense	15,000
Decrease in accounts receivable..	10,000
Decrease in inventory.................	20,000
Increase in notes payable...........	31,000
Decrease in accounts payable	(30,000)
Net cash provided by operating activities	$ 140,000

Cash flows from investing activities:

Cash paid to acquire new buildings	$(125,000)

Cash flows from financing activities:

Cash received from issuance of long-term debt	$ 53,000
Cash received from issuance of common stock	5,000
Payment of cash dividends on common stock	(67,000)
Net cash used for financing activities.........	(9,000)
Net increase in cash for the year	$ 6,000

P9-27. a.

HARRIS, INC.
Balance Sheet
December 31, 2002

Assets

Current assets:

Cash	$ 6,000	
Accounts receivable	67,000	
Merchandise inventory	46,000	
Total current assets		$ 119,000

Noncurrent assets:

Land	27,000	
Buildings	208,000	
Less: Accumulated depreciation	(101,000)	
Total noncurrent assets		134,000
Total assets		$ 253,000

Liabilities and Owners' Equity

Current liabilities:

Short-term debt	$ 12,000	
Notes payable	24,000	
Accounts payable	61,000	
Total current liabilities		$ 97,000
Long-term debt		65,000

Owners' equity:

Common stock, no par	$ 28,000	
Retained earnings	63,000	
Total owners' equity		91,000
Total liabilities and owners' equity		$ 253,000

b.

HARRIS, INC.
Statement of Changes in Retained Earnings
For the Year Ended December 31, 2002

Retained earnings, 1/1/02	$ 55,000
Add: Net income for the year	13,000
Less: Dividends for the year	(5,000)
Retained earnings balance 12/31/02	$ 63,000

Explanatory Notes and Other Financial Information

E10-1. Class discussion can focus on the importance of these items to a reader's full understanding of the company's financial statements (financial position, results of operations, and cash flows).

E10-3. The auditors' opinion is that the identified financial statements *present fairly, in all material respects* (emphasis added), the financial position, results of operations, and cash flows in conformity with generally accepted accounting principles. Thus, the auditor does guarantee that the statements are free of *immaterial* errors (only that they are free of material errors) or that the statements present the financial position, results of operations, and cash flows *perfectly* (only that they present the statements fairly).

E10-5. a. Original earnings per share is $3.12. To reflect a 3 for 1 stock split, divide by 3. Adjusted EPS = **$1.04**

    b. For 2002, 2000 earnings per share as adjusted in 2001 will have to be adjusted again by dividing by 2. Adjusted EPS for 2000, to be reported in 2002 = $1.04 / 2 = **$0.52**

    c. To reflect a 10% stock dividend, divide unadjusted earnings per share by 1.10. Adjusted EPS = $3.12 / 1.10 = **$2.84**

E10-7.

Earnings per share, as restated	$0.60
Multiply by 2 to reflect 2 for 1 stock split	$1.20
Multiply by 1.05 to reflect 5% stock dividend	**$1.26**
Proof: Original earnings per share	$1.26
Adjust for stock split (divide by 2)	$0.63
Adjust for 5% stock dividend (divide by 1.05)	$0.60

P10-9. a. Net revenues in 1992 = **$5,844 million**

    b. Gross profit in 1995 = $16,202 − $7,811 = **$8,391 million**

    c. Difference between operating income and net income in 1997 = $9,887 − $6,945 = **$2,942 million**

P10-9. d. Year(s) in which net income decreased as compared to the previous year = **1994, 1998**

e. Potential obligation under put warrants = **$130 million** *(table, p.20)*

f. Amount of short-term debt = **$230 million** *(table, p.20)*
Amount of long-term debt = **$955 million** *(table, p.20)*

g. Total revenues from unaffiliated customers outside of the Unites States =
$16,649 million *(table, p.28, Total revenues $29,389 less U.S. $12,740)*

h. Amount committed for the construction of property, plant, and equipment =
Approximately $2.5 billion *(p.27)*

i. Amount of available-for-sale securities classified as cash equivalents =
$3,362 million *(p. 21)*

j. Gross profit for the third quarter of 1999 = $7,328 – $3,026 =
$4,302 million *(table, p.37—use September 25 column)*

k. Amount of interest income earned = **$618 million** *(table, p.23)*

P10-11. a.- e. Answers vary depending on the company analyzed.

E11-1. Key data would be the recent (3-5 year) trend in earnings per share, cash dividends per share, market price, and P/E ratio. These data would be in tabular and graphic format.

Market price would be noted weekly. Quarterly and annual data to note are earnings and dividend trends.

The sell/hold/buy decision is based on stock price performance relative to the price objective established from analysis of the above data.

E11-3. *Transaction/event*	*Financial ratio*	+/−	*Explanation*
a. Split the common stock 2 for 1.	Book value per share of common stock.	−	The denominator doubles so the BV/share will be ½ of original.
b. Collected accounts receivable.	Number of days' sales in accounts receivable.	−	Decrease in accounts receivable with no effect on average days' sales.
c. Issued common stock for cash.	Total asset turnover	−	Increase in average total assets with no effect on sales.
d. Sold treasury stock.	Return on equity	−	Increase in average owners' equity with no effect on net income.
e. Accrued interest on a note receivable.	Current ratio	+	Increase in current assets for interest receivable.
f. Sold inventory on account.	Acid-test ratio	+	Numerator increases (inventory turns into accounts receivable).
g. Wrote off an uncollectible account.	Accounts receivable turnover	NE	Net realizable value of accounts receivable is not affected by the write-off entry.
h. Declared a cash dividend.	Dividend yield	+	Dividends per share increase with no determinable effect on market price per share.
i. Incurred operating expenses.	Margin	−	Expenses reduce net income.
j. Sold equipment at a loss.	Earnings per share	+	Losses reduce net income.

P11-5.

INTEL CORPORATION
Common Size Balance Sheet
December 26, 1998

Total current assets	42.8%
Property, plant and equipment, (net)...	36.9
Marketable strategic equity securities and other long-term investments.........	17.0
Goodwill, acquisition-related intangibles, and other assets	3.3
Total assets	100.0%
Total current liabilities.	18.4%
Total noncurrent liabilities *	7.3
Total shareholders' equity.......................	74.3
Total liabilities and shareholders' equity	100.0%

* Includes: long-term debt, deferred tax liabilities, and put warrants.

P11-7. a. Working capital = (current assets – current liabilities) = CA – CL = \$300,000
Current ratio = (current assets / current liabilities) = CA / CL = 2.0

Solution approach:
1) In the current ratio equation, multiply both sides by CL, giving:
 CA = 2CL
2) In the working capital equation, substitute 2CL for CA, giving:
 2CL – CL = \$300,000
 Current liabilities = \$300,000

3) Current assets can be determined as: CA = 2CL = (2 * \$300,000) = \$600,000

 b. Current assets = (Cash + Accounts Receivable + Merchandise Inventory) = \$600,000
 Current liabilities = \$300,000
 Current ratio = 2.0
 Acid-test ratio = 1.5

Solution approach:
1) The difference between the current ratio and the acid-test ratio is that
 Merchandise Inventory is excluded from the numerator of the acid-test ratio.
2) The numerator of the acid test ratio = (CL * 1.5) = (\$300,000 * 1.5) = \$450,000,
 which represents Cash + Accounts Receivable.
3) \$600,000 – \$450,000 = **\$150,000 Merchandise Inventory.**

P11-7. c. *Solution approach:*

The journal entry for collecting an account receivable involves a debit to one current asset (Cash) and a credit to another current asset (Accounts Receivable). Thus, current assets do not change in total, and there is no effect on working capital or the current ratio. **Current ratio = 2.0   Working capital = $300,000**

d. *Solution approach:*

The journal entry for the payment of an account payable involves a debit to a current liability (Accounts Payable) and a credit to a current asset (Cash). Thus, current assets and current liabilities decrease by an equal amount, and there is no effect on working capital. However, the current ratio increases because current assets become proportionately higher than current liabilities.

	Before	*After*
Current assets (A)	$600,000	$500,000
Current liabilities (B)................	300,000	200,000
Working capital (A − B)..........	300,000	**300,000**
Current ratio (A / B)	2.0	**2.5**

e. *Solution approach:*

The journal entries for the sale of inventory would be:

Dr. Cash (included in acid-test numerator)....	$60,000	
Cr. Sales		$60,000
Dr. Cost of Goods Sold...........	50,000	
Cr. Merchandise Inventory (excluded from acid-test numerator) .		50,000

By selling inventory for cash, Arch Company will improve its **acid-test ratio** to **1.7** because a current asset that is included in the acid-test numerator (Cash of $60,000) will replace a current asset that was previously excluded from the acid-test numerator (Merchandise Inventory of $50,000).

Acid-test ratio = $\dfrac{\text{Cash (including temporary cash investments)} + \text{Accounts receivable}}{\text{current liabilities}}$

Before transaction: **After transaction:**

$450,000 / $300,000 = 1.5   ($450,000 + $60,000) / $300,000 = **1.7**

P11-9. a.

	ROI	=	**MARGIN**	x	**TURNOVER**
	$\dfrac{\textbf{NET INCOME}}{\textbf{AVERAGE TOTAL ASSETS}}$	=	$\dfrac{\textbf{NET INCOME}}{\textbf{SALES}}$	x	$\dfrac{\textbf{SALES}}{\textbf{AVERAGE TOTAL ASSETS}}$

P11-9. a. *(continued)*

> 2002 ROI = ($192 / $3,050) * [$3,050 / (($3,090 + $2,811) / 2)]
> = **6.3%** margin * **1.034** turnover = **6.5%**

> 2001 ROI = ($187 / $2,913) * [$2,913 / (($2,455 + $2,811) / 2)]
> = **6.4%** margin * **1.106** turnover = **7.1%**

b. ROE = Net income / Average owners' equity

> 2002 ROE = $192 / (($1,007 + $1,026) / 2) = **18.9%**
> 2001 ROE = $187 / (($918 + $1,026) / 2) = **19.2%**

c.

	2002	*2001*	*2000*
Current assets..	$677	$891	$736
Current liabilities...	(562)	(803)	(710)
Working capital..	**$115**	**$ 88**	**$ 26**
Current ratio (current asset / current liabilities)...............	**1.2**	**1.1**	**1.0**

d. Earnings per share = Net income / Weighted average number of shares outstanding

> 2002 EPS = $192 / 41.3 = **$4.65**
> 2001 EPS = $187 / 46.7 = **$4.00**

e. Price/Earnings ratio = Market price / Earnings per share

> 13 = $??? / $4.65
> Market price = **$60.45**

f. Cash dividends per share = ($50 million total cash dividend / 41.3 million weighted average number of shares outstanding) = **$1.21**

> Dividend yield = ($1.21 cash dividend per share / $60.45 market price per share) = **2%**

g. Dividend payout ratio = ($1.21 dividend per share / $4.65 earnings per share) = **26%**

h. Average days' sales = ($3,050 sales / 365 days) = $8.356 million

> Number of days' sales in accounts receivable = ($309 accounts receivable / $8.356 average day's sales) = **37.0 days**

P11-9. i. Debt ratio = Total liabilities / (Total liabilities + Total owners' equity)

12/31/02 Debt ratio = ($562 + $1,521) / $3,090 = **67.4%**
12/31/01 Debt ratio = ($803 + $982) / $2,811 = **63.5%**

Debt/equity ratio = Total liabilities / Total owners' equity

12/31/02 Debt/equity ratio = ($562 + $1,521) / $1,007 = **207%**
12/31/01 Debt/equity ratio = ($803 + $982) / $1,026 = **174%**

j. Times interest earned = Operating income / Interest expense

For 2002: = $296 / $84 = **3.5 times**
For 2001: = $310 / $65 = **4.8 times**

k. A young, single professional would probably be more interested in potential growth of capital rather than current dividend income, and would probably be willing to invest in a stock that represented a relatively risky investment. Based on these criteria, the significant growth in earnings per share and the relatively high financial leverage could make this stock an attractive, though risky, potential investment.

The liquidity of the company is relatively low, based on an "average" current ratio of 1.0. Without further information about the composition of the current asset and current liability accounts, it is difficult to assess the firm's liquidity. The number of days' sales in accounts receivable indicates that the accounts receivable are relatively current, assuming that the credit terms are net 30.

The company's ROI is relatively low, and the two-year trend is down. This would be a major concern, and the reasons for this situation would be sought. The price/earnings ratio of 13 is typical for a firm with a falling ROI; the fact that the P/E ratio has remained within the "normal" range may indicate that future earnings prospects for this firm are fairly strong.

P11-11. a. ROI = Net income / Average total assets

Dow Jones	**McGraw-Hill**
= $272 / (($1,484 + $1,531) / 2) =	= $426 / (($3,788 + $4,088) /2) =
= $272 / $1,508 = **18.0%**	= $426 / $3,938 = **10.8%**

Note: Total assets at the end of the year is equal to ending liabilities *plus* ending stockholders' equity. For Dow Jones, $977 + $554 = $1,531. For McGraw-Hill, $2,397 + $1,691 = $4,088.

P11-11. a. *(continued)*

ROE = Net income / Average stockholders' equity

Dow Jones	***McGraw-Hill***
= $272 / (($509 + $554) / 2)	= $426 / (($1,552 + $1,691) /2)
= $272 / $531.5 = **51.2%**	= $426 / $1,621.5 = **26.3%**

Note: Total stockholders' equity at the beginning of the year is equal to beginning assets *minus* beginning liabilities. For Dow Jones, $1,484 – $975 = $509. For McGraw-Hill, $3,788 – $2,236 = $1,552.

b. Yes. It appears that Dow-Jones uses significantly more financial leverage than does McGraw-Hill. The magnification effect of Dow Jones' ROE (of 51.2%) relative to its ROI (of 18.0%) is approximately 284%; that is, ROE is 284% greater than ROI. For Dow Jones, although the spread between ROE (of 26.3%) and ROI (of 10.8%) is much smaller, the magnification effect of financial leverage (of 243%) is also quite significant.

c. Debt ratio = Total liabilities / (Total liabilities + Total stockholders' equity)

Dow Jones	***McGraw-Hill***
= $977 / ($977 + $554) = **63.8%**	= $2,397 / ($2,397 + $1,691) = **58.6%**

Debt/equity ratio = Total liabilities / Total stockholders' equity

Dow Jones	***McGraw-Hill***
= $977 / $554 = **1.76, or 176%**	= $2,397 / $1,691 = **1.42, or 142%**

d. The debt and debt/equity ratios calculated in part *c* make sense relative to the student's expectations formed in part *b*. As expected, Dow Jones is somewhat more leveraged than is McGraw-Hill. Thus, profitability analysis (ROI and ROE) can give important signals concerning financial leverage measures (debt and debt/equity). The opposite is also true (which could easily be demonstrated by reversing the order of parts *a* and *c* in this problem). That is, the more leveraged a firm is, the greater the expected magnification of ROE relative to ROI.

P11-13. a.1. Income statement (or statement of operations).
    2. Net income (or net earnings).
    3. Earnings per share of common stock.
    4. Statement of changes in owners' (or stockholders') equity.
    5. Retained earnings.
    6. Owners' (or stockholders') equity.
    7. Working capital.
    8. Owners' (or stockholders') equity.

b. 1.

ROI	=	MARGIN	x	TURNOVER
$\dfrac{\text{OPERATING INCOME}}{\text{AVERAGE TOTAL ASSETS}}$	=	$\dfrac{\text{OPERATING INCOME}}{\text{SALES}}$	x	$\dfrac{\text{SALES}}{\text{AVERAGE TOTAL ASSETS}}$

Margin = ($498 operating profit / $8,251 sales) = **6.0%**

Turnover = Sales / ((Total assets less current liabilities + Current liabilities) / 2)
    = $8,251 / [(($4,873 + $2,758) + ($4,289 + $2,472)) / 2] = **1.15**

ROI = (6.0% Margin * 1.15 Turnover) = **6.9%**

  2. ROE = (Net income / Average owners' equity) = (Profit / Average ownership)
    = $350 / (($3,565 + $3,149) / 2) = **10.4%**

c. 1. Average day's sales = ($8,251 annual sales / 365 days) = $22.6 million

    Number of days' sales in accounts receivable = ($2,174 accounts receivable /
    $22.6 average day's sales) = **96.2 days**

  2. Inventory turnover = Cost of goods sold / Average inventory
    = $6,523 / (($1,323 + $1,211) / 2) = **5.1 times**

  3. Plant and equipment turnover = Sales / Average plant and equipment
    = Sales / ((Buildings, machinery, and equipment + Land) / 2)
    = $8,251 / [(($2,467 + $96) + ($2,431 + $97)) / 2] = **3.2 times**

d. 1. Debt/equity ratio = ($1,287 long-term debt / $3,565 ownership) = **36.1%**

  2. Debt ratio = ($1,287 long-term debt / ($1,287 long-term debt
    + $3,565 ownership)) = **26.5%**

  3. Times interest earned = (Earnings before interest and taxes / Interest expense)
    = ($498 operating profit / $209) = **2.4 times**

P11-13. e. 1. Price/earning ratio = (Market price per share / Earning per share)
= ($42.00 / $3.51 profit per share of common stock after extraordinary tax benefit) = **12.0**

2. Dividend payout ratio = (Dividends per share / Earning per share)
= ($0.50 dividends paid per share of common stock / $3.51 profit per share of common stock after extraordinary tax benefit) = **14.2%**

3. Dividend yield = (Dividends per share / Market price per share)
= ($0.50 dividends paid per share of common stock / $42.00) = **1.2%**

Managerial Accounting and Cost-Volume-Profit Analysis

E12-1.

	Variable	Fixed
Wages of assembly-line workers	X	_____
Depreciation--plant equipment	_____	X
Glue and thread..	X	_____
Shipping costs	X	_____
Raw materials handling costs	X	_____
Salary of public relations manager	_____	X
Production run setup costs	X	_____
Plant utilities..	X	X
Electricity cost of retail stores	X	X
Research and development expenses	X	X

Note: The last three items are each likely to have a mixed cost behavior pattern.

E12-3.

a. Total cost = ($320 fixed cost + ($0.14 variable cost per mile * 1,529 miles)) = **$534.06**

b. No, it would not be meaningful to calculate an average cost per mile, because that would involve unitizing the fixed expenses, and they do not behave on a per mile basis. Whatever average cost per mile were calculated would be valid only for the number of miles used in the calculation. An average cost for any other number of miles driven would be different, because the fixed expenses per mile would decrease for each additional mile driven.

E12-5.   *Note to Student:* The purpose of this assignment is to help you to build an understanding of cost-volume-profit relationships by solving for the 'missing pieces of the puzzles.' In this regard, it may be helpful to insert a *Contribution Margin* column, or to rearrange the data using the expanded contribution margin model.

Answer:	Sales	Variable Costs	Contribution Margin Ratio	Fixed Costs	Operating Income (Loss)
Firm A	$320,000	**$217,600**	32%	**$64,100**	$38,300
Firm B	**655,000**	465,050	**29%**	118,000	71,950
Firm C	134,000	**99,160**	26%	36,700	**(1,860)**
Firm D	**73,750**	59,000	20%	**19,670**	(4,920)

Calculations:

    Firm A   VC = Sales * (1 – CM%) = $320,000 * 68% = **$217,600**

                     CM = Sales – VC = $320,000 – $217,600 = $102,400

                     or CM = Sales * CM% = $320,000 * 32% = $102,400

E12-5. *(continued)*

FC = CM – Operating Income = $102,400 – $38,300 = **$64,100**
or FC = (Sales * CM%) – Operating Income = ($320,000 * 32%) –
$38,300 = **$64,100**

Firm B   CM = FC + Operating Income = $118,000 + $71,950 = $189,950
Sales = CM + VC = $189,950 + $465,050 = **$655,000**
CM% = CM / Sales = $189,950 / $655,000 = **29%**

Firm C   VC = Sales * (1 – CM%) = $134,000 * 74% = **$99,160**
CM = Sales – VC = $134,000 – $99,160 = $34,840
or CM = Sales * CM% = $134,000 * 26% = $34,840
Operating Loss = CM – FC = $34,840 – $36,700 = **$(1,860)**

Firm D   Sales = VC / (1 – CM%) = $59,000 / 80% = **$73,750**
CM = Sales – VC = $73,750 – $59,000 = $14,750
or CM = Sales * CM% = $73,750 * 20% = $14,750
FC = CM + Operating (Loss) = $14,750 + $4,920 = **$19,670**

E12-7.

a.   Use the model, enter the known data, and solve for the unknown.

	Per Unit	*	Volume	=	Total	%
Revenue	$?					100%
Variable Expense	7.80					65%
Contribution Margin	$?	*		=	$	35%

Variable expenses = 65% of selling price. Selling price = $7.80 / 65% = **$12.00**

b.

	Per Unit	*	Volume	=	Total	%
Revenue	$12.00					100%
Variable Expense	7.80					65%
Contribution Margin	$ 4.20	*	?	=	$?	35%
Fixed Expense					(15,000)	
Operating Income					$ 6,000	

Total contribution margin = ($15,000 + $6,000) = $21,000. Total contribution margin
divided by the contribution margin per unit of $4.20 gives **5,000 units** of the new
product that would have to be sold to increase operating income by $6,000.

E12-9.

a.

	Per Unit	*	Volume	=	Total	%
Revenue	$1.25					100%
Variable Expense	0.35					28%
Contribution Margin	$0.90	*	400	=	$ 360	72%
Fixed Expense					(120)	
Operating income from increased volume					$ 240	
Variable expenses of 600 cones given away, @ $0.35					(210)	
Net increase in operating income					$ 30	

b. Yes. Not only does the promotion itself result in increased operating income, but also it is likely that customers will purchase some other products (e.g., food and/or beverages) on which additional contribution margin will be earned.

P12-11.

a. ***Solution approach:*** First, calculate variable cost per unit in February and use the same per unit cost for April. Second, fixed cost will be the same for each month. Third, with knowledge of total costs for April, and variable and fixed costs for April, solve for mixed costs for April.

	February	April
Activity	5,000 units	8,000 units
Costs:		
Variable ($10,000 / 5,000 units = $2 per unit)	$10,000	$16,000
Fixed (same total amount each month)	30,000	30,000
Mixed (Total costs − (Variable + Fixed))......	20,000	**24,500**
Total	$60,000	$70,500

b.

$$\text{Variable rate} = (\text{High \$} - \text{Low \$}) / (\text{High units} - \text{Low units})$$
$$= (\$24,500 - \$20,000) / (8,000 - 5,000)$$
$$= \$4,500 / 3,000 = \textbf{\$1.50 per unit}$$

$$\text{Total mixed cost} = \text{Fixed cost} + \text{Variable cost}$$
$$\$24,500 = ? + (\$1.50 * 8,000 \text{ units})$$
$$? = \textbf{\$12,500}$$

$$\text{Cost formula} = \text{Fixed cost} + (\text{Variable rate} * \text{Volume})$$
$$= \textbf{\$12,500 + \$1.50 per unit}$$

Proof at 5,000 units: Mixed cost = $12,500 + ($1.50 * 5,000 units) = $20,000

P12-13.

a.
Revenues (8,000 units * $4 per unit)		$32,000
Variable expenses:		
Cost of goods sold (8,000 units * $ 2.10 per unit)	$16,800	
Selling expenses (8,000 unit * $0.10 per unit)	800	
Administrative expenses (8,000 units * $0.20 per unit)	1,600	
Total variable expenses		19,200
Contribution margin		$12,800
Fixed expenses:		
Cost of goods sold	$6,000	
Selling expenses	1,200	
Administrative expenses..................................	4,000	
Total fixed expenses		11,200
Operating income		$ 1,600

b. Contribution margin per unit = Total CM / Volume = $12,800 / 8,000 units = **$1.60**
Alternative approach:
CM per unit = Selling price per unit – Variable expense per unit
   = $4.00 – $2.40 = **$1.60 per unit**
Contribution margin ratio = CM / Revenues = $12,800 / $32,000 = **40%**
Alternative approach:
CM ratio = CM per unit / Selling price per unit = $1.60 / $4.00 = **40%**

c. 1. **Volume of 12,000 units:**

	Per Unit	*	*Volume*	=	*Total*	*%*
Revenue	$4.00					100%
Variable Expense	2.40					60%
Contribution Margin	$1.60	*	12,000	=	$19,200	40%
Fixed Expense					(11,200)	
Operating Income					$ 8,000	

Alternative approach: 4,000 more units sold @ $1.60 CM per unit = $6,400 increase in contribution margin and operating income. Present operating income is $1,600, so new operating income will be $8,000.

2. **Volume of 4,000 units:**

	Per Unit	*	*Volume*	=	*Total*	*%*
Revenue	$4.00					100%
Variable Expense	2.40					60%
Contribution Margin	$1.60	*	4,000	=	$ 6,400	40%
Fixed Expense (no change)					(11,200)	
Operating Loss					$(4,800)	

Alternative approach: Operating income decreases by $6,400 (4,000 units * $1.60 per unit) from present operating income of $1,600, causing an operating loss of $4,800.

P12-13. *(continued)*

d. 1. Use the contribution margin ratio of 40%. Revenue increase of $12,000 causes a $4,800 increase (40% * $12,000) in contribution margin and operating income. Operating income = $1,600 + $4,800 = **$6,400**

2. Revenue decrease of $7,000 causes a $2,800 decrease (40% * $7,000) in contribution margin and operating income. Operating income changes to a loss = $1,600 − $2,800 = **$(1,200)**

P12-15.

a.

Sales	$65,000
Variable expenses (80% * $65,000)	(52,000)
Contribution margin (20% * $65,000)	$13,000
Fixed expenses	(18,000)
Operating loss	$(5,000)

Note: Operating loss remains the same, so Fixed expenses = ($13,000 Contribution margin + $5,000 Operating loss).

b.

Increase in sales (30% * $65,000)	$19,500
Contribution margin ratio	20%
Increase in contribution margin	$ 3,900
Previous operating loss	(5,000)
Adjusted operating loss	$(1,100)

Operating loss = $(5,000) + $3,900 = **$(1,100)**. The increase in contribution margin is also a decrease in the operating loss, because fixed expenses do not change.

c. At break-even, contribution margin = fixed expenses = $18,000
Contribution margin = (20% contribution margin ratio * ??? sales) = $18,000
Sales = ($18,000 fixed expenses / 20% CM ratio) = $90,000 at break-even.

P12-17.

a.

	Per Unit	*	*Volume*	=	*Total*
Revenue	$15				
Variable Expense	9				
Contribution Margin	$ 6	*	?	=	$ 27,000
Fixed Expense					(27,000)
Operating Income					$ 0

At the break-even point, total contribution margin must equal total fixed expenses. Break-even volume = ($6 contribution margin per unit * ??? volume) = $27,000 Thus, break-even volume = **4,500 units** Total revenue = (4,500 units * $15 per unit) = **$67,500**

Alternative approach: $27,000 / 40% contribution margin ratio = **$67,500**

P12-17. *(continued)*

b.

	Per Unit	*	Volume	=	Total
Revenue	$15				
Variable Expense	9				
Contribution Margin	$ 6	*	5,400	=	$32,400
Fixed Expense					(27,000)
Operating Income					**$ 5,400**

c.

	Per Unit	*	Volume	=	Total
Revenue	$13				
Variable Expense	9				
Contribution Margin	$ 4	*	8,400	=	$33,600
Fixed Expense					(27,000)
Operating Income					**$ 6,600**

d. Does the increase in volume move fixed expenses into a new relevant range? Are variable expenses really linear?

e.

	Per Unit	*	Volume	=	Total
Revenue	$16				
Variable Expense	9				
Contribution Margin	$ 7	*	5,400	=	$37,800
Fixed Expense					(33,000)
Operating Income					**$ 4,800**

f. 1. *Volume of 5,400 units per month:*

	Per Unit	*	Volume	=	Total
Revenue	$15.00				
Variable Expense	9.80				
Contribution Margin	$ 5.20	*	5,400	=	$28,080
Fixed Expense #					(22,800)
Operating Income					**$ 5,280**

# Current fixed expenses...		$27,000
Decrease in fixed expenses (2 salespersons @ $2,500)		(5,000)
Increase in fixed expenses (2 salespersons @ $400)		800
Adjusted fixed expenses		$22,800

2. *Volume of 6,000 units per month:*

	Per Unit	*	Volume	=	Total
Revenue	$15.00				
Variable Expense	9.80				
Contribution Margin	$ 5.20	*	6,000	=	$31,200
Fixed Expense					(22,800)
Operating Income					**$ 8,400**

P12-17. *(continued)*

	Per Unit	*	Volume	=	Total
Revenue	$15				
Variable Expense	9				
Contribution Margin	$6	*	6,000	=	$36,000
Fixed Expense					(28,000)
Operating Income					**$ 8,000**

The sales force compensation plan change results in $400 more operating income than does the plan to increase advertising.

P12-19.

a. & b.

Current Operation:	*Luxury*	*Economy*	*Total*
Revenue	$20 * 10,000 = $200,000	$12 * 20,000 = $240,000	$440,000
Variable Expense	8	7	
Contribution Margin	$12 * 10,000 = $120,000	$ 5 * 20,000 = $100,000	**$220,000**
Fixed Expense			(70,000)
Operating Income			**$150,000**

Total contribution margin = $120,000 + $100,000 = **$220,000**
Average contribution margin ratio = $220,000 / $440,000 = **50%**
Operating income = $220,000 − $70,000 = **$150,000**

c. Break-even point in sales dollars = Fixed expenses / Contribution margin ratio
   = $70,000 / 50% = **$140,000**

d. Because sales mix might change. For example, if the company sold *only* the economy model, total contribution margin would equal the economy model contribution margin ratio ($5 / $12 = 41.666%) multiplied by the current break-even point in sales dollars of $140,000, which equals $58,333. Note that this amount is less than the $70,000 of fixed expenses, so the firm would have to generate a higher sales volume to break even. The opposite would be true if the company sold *only* the luxury model—with a contribution margin ratio of 60% ($12 / $20), total contribution margin would be $84,000 ($140,000 * 60%), and the break-even point in sales dollars would fall from $140,000 to $116,667 ($70,000 fixed expenses / 60% contribution margin ratio).

e. *Proposed Expansion:*

	Luxury	*Economy*	*Value*	*Total*
Rev.	$20 * 6,000 = $120,000	$12 * 17,000 = $204,000	$15 * 8,000 = $120,000	$444,000
VE	8	7	8	
CM	$12 * 6,000 = $ 72,000	$ 5 * 17,000 = $ 85,000	$ 7 * 8,000 = $ 56,000	$213,000
FE				(84,000)
OI				**$129,000**

f. No. Based on this data analysis, adding the Value model would result in lower total operating income by $21,000 ($150,000 current operation versus $129,000 proposed).

P12-19. *(continued)*

g. No. Although 2,000 more units of the Value model would increase total contribution margin and operating income by $14,000 (2,000 units @ $ 7 CM per unit), operating income would rise only to $143,000, which is still less than under the current operation.

P12-21.

a.

	Per Unit	*	*Volume*	=	*Total*	*%*
Revenue	$32					100.0%
Variable Expense	20					62.5%
Contribution Margin	$12	*	4,100	=	$49,200	37.5%
Fixed Expense					(43,200)	
Operating Income					**$ 6,000**	

b.

	Per Unit	*	*Volume*	=	*Total*	*%*
Revenue	$32					100.0%
Variable Expense	20					62.5%
Contribution Margin	$12	*	?	=	$43,200	37.5%
Fixed Expense					(43,200)	
Operating Income					$ 0	

Break-even volume = $43,200 / $12 per unit = **3,600 units**
Break-even revenues = 3,600 units * $32 per unit = **$115,200**

c. 1.

	Per Unit	*	*Volume*	=	*Total*	*%*
Revenue	$32					100.00%
Variable Expense	14					43.75%
Contribution Margin	$18	*	4,100	=	$73,800	56.25%
Fixed Expense					(67,800)	
Operating Income					**$ 6,000**	

2.

	Per Unit	*	*Volume*	=	*Total*	*%*
Revenue	$32					100.00%
Variable Expense	14					43.75%
Contribution Margin	$18	*	?	=	$67,800	56.25%
Fixed Expense					(67,800)	
Operating Income					$ 0	

Break-even volume = $67,800 / $18 = **3,767 units** (rounded)
Break-even revenues = 3,767 units * $32 = **$120,533** (rounded)

3. As sales volume moves above the break-even point, contribution margin and operating income will increase by a greater amount per unit sold than under the old cost structure.

4. The new cost structure has much more risk, because if sales volume declines, the impact on contribution margin and operating income will be greater than under the old cost structure.

E13-1.

Business Function	Cost Item	Answer
a. Research & Development	1. Purchase of raw materials	c
b. Design	2. Advertising	d
c. Production	3. Salary of research scientists	a
d. Marketing	4. Shipping expenses	e
e. Distribution	5. Reengineering of product assembly process	b
f. Customer Service	6. Replacement parts for warranty repairs	f
	7. Manufacturing supplies	c
	8. Sales commissions	d
	9. Purchase of CAD (Computer Aided Design) software	b
	10. Salary of Web site designer	d

E13-3.

	Product Direct	Indirect	Period	Variable	Fixed
Wages of assembly-line workers...	x			x	
Depreciation–plant equipment ...		x			x
Glue and thread		x		x	
Shipping costs........................			x	x	
Raw materials handling costs......		x		x	
Salary of public relations manager			x		x
Production run setup costs		x		x	
Plant utilities		x		x	x
Electricity cost of retail stores......			x	x	x
Research and development expenses			x	x	x

Note: The last three items are each likely to have a mixed cost behavior pattern.

E13-5.
a. *Raw material:* cotton/ wool/ rayon used for jersey, or material used for team emblems.
b. *Direct labor:* wages of production-line machine operator.
c. *Variable manufacturing overhead:* plant utilities costs, or indirect materials (i.e., thread).
d. *Fixed manufacturing overhead:* depreciation of machinery, or property taxes on plant.
e. *Fixed administrative expense:* salaries of administrative officers.
f. *Fixed indirect selling expense:* advertising costs.
g. *Variable, direct selling expense:* shipping costs.

E13-7.

    a.   Predetermined overhead application rate
        = ($408,750 estimated total overhead cost / 54,500 estimated direct labor hours)
        = **$7.50 per direct labor hour.**

    b.   *Total cost for 750 coffee mugs produced:*

Raw materials	$ 810
Direct labor (90 direct labor hours * $9.50 per hour)	855
Overhead (90 direct labor hours * $7.50 predetermined rate)..............	675
Total manufacturing cost	$ 2,340

        Cost per coffee mug produced = ($2,340 total cost / 750 mugs)
        = **$3.12 per coffee mug.**

    c.   Cost of coffee mugs sold = (530 mugs * $3.12 per mug) = **$1,653.60**
        Cost of coffee mugs in inventory = (220 mugs * $3.12 per mug) = **$686.40**

E13-9.

    a.   9,000 machine hours * $12.70 per machine hour = **$114,300 budgeted overhead.**

    b.

Actual overhead incurred	$121,650
Applied overhead (9,100 machine hours* $12.70 per machine hour)	(115,570)
Underapplied overhead	**$ 6,080**

    c.   The overapplied or underapplied overhead for the year is normally transferred to cost of goods sold in the income statement. Since most products made during the year are sold during the same year, manufacturing overhead costs are assumed to relate primarily to the products sold. However, if the over- or underapplied overhead is material in dollar amount, then it may be allocated between work-in-process, finished goods, and cost of goods sold, based on respective year-end balances.

E13-11.

    Total cost for 530 ties produced:

Raw materials	$1,950
Direct labor (75 direct labor hours)...	840
Overhead applied based on raw materials ($1,950 * 140%)	2,730
Overhead applied based on direct labor hours (75 hours * $7.20)	540
Total manufacturing cost..	$6,060

    Cost per tie produced = $6,060 / 530 units = **$11.43 per unit** (rounded)

P13-13.

a.
Absorption cost per sweater	$11.60
Less: Fixed manufacturing overhead per sweater ($22,500 / 9,000).........	(2.50)
Variable cost per sweater	**$ 9.10**

b. 1,600 sweaters * $2.50 = $4,000 more cost released to the income statement this month under absorption costing than under variable costing. Thus, cost of goods sold under variable costing will be $4,000 lower than under absorption.

c. Total cost = Fixed cost + (variable rate * activity)
   = $22,500 + ($9.10 * number of sweaters)

P13-15.

a. Total manufacturing cost = (Direct materials + Direct labor + Manufacturing overhead)

Direct materials		$3,500,000
Direct labor (160,000 hours * $20 per hour)		3,200,000
Manufacturing overhead:		
Materials handling ($1.50 per part * 275,000 parts used)	$ 412,500	
Milling and grinding ($11.00 per machine hour * 95,000 hours)..	1,045,000	
Assembly and inspection ($5.00 per labor hour * 160,000 hours).	800,000	
Testing ($3.00 per unit * 50,000 units tested).....................	150,000	2,407,500
Total manufacturing cost...		**$9,107,500**

Cost per unit produced and tested = $9,107,500 / 50,000 units = **$182.15 per unit.**

b. The activity based costing approach is likely to provide better information for manufacturing managers because overhead costs are applied based on the activities that *cause* the incurrence of cost (i.e., cost drivers). Thus, management attention will be directed to the critical activities that can be controlled to improve the firm's operating performance. ABC systems also produce more accurate product costing information, which can lead to better decision-making.

P13-17.

a.
Variable manufacturing costs:	
Raw materials	$ 62,100
Direct labor	16,500
Variable manufacturing overhead................................	11,250
Total variable costs	$ 89,850
Fixed manufacturing overhead...................................	18,000
Total manufacturing costs....................................	$107,850

Variable cost per rod = $89,850 / 15,000 = **$5.99 each**
Absorption cost per rod = $107,850 / 15,000 = **$7.19 each**

P13-17. *(continued)*

b. The fixed cost per rod is $7.19 - $5.99 = $1.20.
    This can also be computed as: $18,000 / 15,000 = $1.20.
    The total fixed cost associated with the 300 fishing rods in inventory is:
    300 * $1.20 = $360.

    This amount would be included in ending inventory under absorption costing, but
    would be included in cost of goods sold under variable costing. Thus, under variable
    costing, operating income would be $360 less than under absorption costing.

c. Total cost = $18,000 + $5.99 per fishing rod produced.
    The cost of making 200 more units = 200 * $5.99 = **$1,198**

P13-19.

a.

Raw materials	$ 33,100
Direct labor	65,200
Manufacturing overhead	44,800
Cost of goods manufactured	**$143,100**

Cost per unit = $143,100 / 5,300 = **$27**

b. Cost of goods sold = $27 * 4,800 = **$129,600**

c. The difference between cost of goods manufactured and cost of goods sold
    is in the finished goods inventory account on the balance sheet. Since
    more units were produced (5,300) than sold (4,800), the finished goods
    account will increase by $13,500 ($27 per unit * 500 units), and cost of
    goods sold will be $13,500 less than cost of goods manufactured.

d.

Kimane, Ltd.
Income Statement
For the month of November

Sales	$244,800
Cost of goods sold	(129,600)
Gross profit	$115,200
Selling and administrative expenses	(46,100)
Operating income	$ 69,100
Interest expense	(9,100)
Income before taxes	$ 60,000
Income tax expense	(18,000)
Net income	$ 42,000

P13-21.

a. *Note:* This problem does not require a formal statement of cost of goods manufactured; the requirements can be solved using a "T" account approach.

Raw materials:

Inventory, Sept. 30	$ 33,500	
Purchases during October	123,900	
Raw materials available for use	157,400	
Less: Inventory, Oct. 31..	(27,600)	
Cost of raw materials used......................................		$129,800
Direct labor cost incurred.......................................		312,200
Manufacturing overhead applied		192,300
Total manufacturing costs, October		$634,300
Add: Work-in-process, Sept. 30		71,300
Less: Work-in-process, Oct. 31		(64,800)
Cost of goods manufactured, October		**$640,800**

b.

Finished goods, Sept. 30	$ 47,200
Cost of goods manufactured......................................	640,800
Cost of goods available for sale	$688,000
Less: Finished goods, Oct. 31	(41,900)
Cost of goods sold	**$646,100**

Cost Analysis for Planning

E14-1.

a. Use the cost of goods sold model, and work from the bottom up and then top down to calculate production:

	medallions
Beginning inventory...	1,000
Goods available for sale	?
Less: Ending inventory...	(800)
Quantity sold..	2,000

Goods available for sale = 2,000 + 800 = 2,800 medallions
Production = 2,800 − 1,000 = **1,800 medallions**

b. Use the same approach, but notice that quantity used is a function of quantity produced from the production budget. Each medallion requires 2/3 of a yard of ribbon.

	yards
Beginning inventory...	50
Purchases	?
Raw materials available for use	?
Less: Ending inventory...	(20)
Raw materials used in production (2/3 * 1,800 medallions)...	1,200

Raw materials available for use = 1,200 + 20 = 1,220 yards
Purchases = 1,220 − 50 = **1,170 yards**

E14-3.

a. Use the raw material inventory/usage model:

	Quarter I	Quarter II
Beginning inventory	5,000	9,000
Add: Purchases	?	?
Raw materials available for use	?	?
Less: Ending inventory (25% of next quarter's usage).........	(9,000)	(5,500)
Usage (2 ounces * number of gallons of product to be produced)..	20,000	36,000

	Quarter I	Quarter II
Working backwards (up the model):		
Raw materials available for use	29,000	41,500
Purchases (subtract beginning inventory)......................	**24,000**	**32,500**

b. Inventory provides a "cushion" for delivery delays or production needs in excess of the production forecast.

E14-5.

	May	*June*	*July*	*August*
Sales forecast.............................	$240,000	$280,000	$300,000	$350,000
Cash collections:				
30% of current month's sales			$ 90,000	$105,000
50% of prior month's sales			140,000	150,000
18% of second prior month's sales			43,200	50,400
Total cash collections budget			**$273,200**	**$305,400**

E14-7.

a.
Worktype 1 (0.15 hours @ $12.30 per hour)	$ 1.845
Worktype 2 (0.30 hours @ $10.90 per hour)	3.270
Worktype 3 (0.60 hours @ $19.50 per hour)	11.700
Total direct labor cost per pedestal	**$16.815**

b. No, because the engineer developed ideal standards. It is unlikely that the standards would be met in practice, and they would not provide positive motivation or result in accurate costing.

E14-9.

a.
Raw material cost...	$2.83 per bushel
Direct labor and variable overhead	0.42 per bushel
Fixed overhead...	0.35 per bushel
Total absorption cost	**$3.60 per bushel**

Each bushel yields 15 pounds of product.
Cost per pound = $3.60 / 15 = **$0.24 per pound.**

b. This cost per pound is not very useful for management planning and control because it includes unitized fixed expenses, which do not behave on a per unit basis.

P14-11.

	July	*August*	*September*
Sales forecast	$250,000	$220,000	$310,000
Cost of sales @ 54%	135,000	118,800	167,400
Purchases budget:			
Beginning inventory	$410,000	$356,400	
Purchases...	?	?	
Cost of merchandise available for sale	?	?	
Less: Ending inventory (300% * next			
month's cost of goods sold)	(356,400)	(502,200)	
Cost of goods sold	$135,000	$118,800	

P14.11. *(continued)*

Cost of merchandise available for sale =
(Cost of goods sold + Ending inventory) $491,400 $621,000
Purchases = (Cost of merchandise available
for sale – Beginning inventory) ....   **$ 81,400**   **$264,600**

P14-13.

a.

	September	*October*
Sales forecast	$42,000	$54,000
Purchases budget...	37,800	44,000
Operating expense budget	10,500	12,800
Beginning cash	**$40,000**	
Cash receipts:		
August 31 accounts receivable	20,000	
September sales...	0	
Total cash receipts	**$20,000**	
Cash disbursements:		
August 31 accounts payable and accrued expenses	$24,000	
September purchases (75% * $37,800).....................	28,350	
September operating expenses (75% * $10,500)	7,875	
Total cash disbursements	**$60,225**	
Ending cash..	**$ (225)**	

b. QB Sportswear's management should try to accelerate the collection of accounts receivable, slow down the payment of accounts payable and accrued expenses, and/or negotiate a bank loan. If sales growth continues at a very high rate, they probably will need to secure some permanent financing through sale of bonds or stock.

P14-15. *Answer (and one possible numbered sequence of solving the problem):*

	July	*August*	*September*	*Total*
Cash balance, beginning	$ 26	9. **$ 20**	10. **$ 20**	$ 26
Add collections from customers ...	1. **68**	107	11. **136**	17. **311**
Total cash available..............	94	8. **127**	156	337

P14-15.	(continued)	July	August	September	Total
	Less disbursements:				
	Purchase of inventory	3. **50**	60	48	18. **158**
	Operating expenses	30	7. **39**	16. **24**	19. **93**
	Capital additions	34	8	15. **2**	44
	Payment of dividends	-	-	14. **9**	9
	Total disbursements	2. **114**	107	83	304
	Excess (deficiency) of cash				
	available over disbursements ...	(20)	6. **20**	73	20. **33**
	Borrowings	5. **40**	-	-	21. **40**
	Repayments (including interest).	-	-	13. **41**	22. **41**
	Cash balance, ending	4. **$ 20**	$ 20	12. **$ 32**	$ 32

Solution approach:
1. $94 – $26 = **$68**,
2. $94 + 20 (deficiency of cash available) = **$114**,
3. $114 – $30 – $34 = **$50**,
4. Minimum month-end balance,
5. $20 + 20 (deficiency of cash available) = **$40**,
6. Equal to ending cash balance for August because there were no borrowings or repayments during the month.
7. $107 – $60 – $8 = **$39**,
8. $107 + $20 (excess of cash available) = **$127**,
9. $127 – $107 = **$20** (or **$20** ending balance from July carried forward),
10. Ending cash balance from August is carried forward to beginning cash balance of September = **$20**,
11. $156 – $20 = **$136**,
12. Ending cash balance for the third quarter is the ending cash balance for September = **$32**,
13. $73 – $32 = **$41**,
14. Total dividends = **$9**, and no dividends were paid in July and August,
15. $44 total capital additions – $34 – $8 = **$2**,
16. $83 – $48 – $2 – $9 = **$24**,
17. $337 – $26 = **$311**,
18. Total purchases (across) = $50 + $60 + $48 = **$158**,
19. Total operating, expenses (across) = $30 + $39 + $24 = **$93**,
    or $304 – $158 – $44 – $9 = **$93**,
20. $337 – $304 = **$33**,
21. Borrowings from July,
22. Repayments in September.

P14-17.

a.

	April	*May*	*June*	*Total*
Expected sales in units	7,000	10,000	8,000	25,000
Selling price per unit	$40	$40	$40	$40
Total sales	**$280,000**	**$400,000**	**$320,000**	**$1,000,000**

b.

Cash collections from:	*April*	*May*	*June*	*Total*
March sales	$132,000[a]			$132,000
April sales	112,000	$154,000		266,000
May sales		160,000	$220,000	380,000
June sales			128,000	128,000
Total cash collections	**$244,000**	**$314,000**	**$348,000**	**$906,000**

[a] Sales from February and all prior months would have been fully collected (or written off) by the end of March. Thus, the $132,000 net realizable value of accounts receivable represents the 55% of March sales that will be collected in April (6,000 units sold in March * $40 * 55% = $132,000).

	April	*May*	*June*	*Total*
c. Beginning inventory of				
finished goods	3,500	5,000	4,000	3,500
Units to be produced............	**8,500**	**9,000**	**8,500**	**26,000**
Goods available for sale	12,000	14,000	12,500	29,500
Desired ending inventory of				
finished goods (50% of next				
month's budgeted sales)	(5,000)	(4,000)	(4,500)	(4,500)
Quantity of goods sold	7,000	10,000	8,000	25,000

Note: In the total column, the beginning and ending inventory figures represent the number of units on hand at April 1, 2002 and June 30, 2002, respectively. Thus, the "goods available for sale" line does not add across.

d.

	April	*May*	*June*	*Total*
Beginning inventory of				
raw materials	10,200	10,800	10,200	10,200
Purchases of raw materials	**26,100**	**26,400**	**24,300**	**76,800**
Raw materials available for use.	36,300	37,200	34,500	87,000
Desired ending inventory of				
raw materials (40% of next				
month's estimated usage)[b]	(10,800)	(10,200)	(9,000)[c]	(9,000)
Quantity of raw materials to be				
used in production[d]	25,500	27,000	25,500	78,000

[b] Next month's "units to be produced" (see answer to part c) is multiplied by three pounds to determine raw material requirements, which is then multiplied by 40%.

P14-17. *(continued)*

(c) To determine the desired ending inventory of raw materials for June, the "units to be produced" in July must be determined. This is done in the same manner as shown in the answer to part *c* for April, May, and June:

	July
Beginning inventory of finished goods (carried over from June)	4,500
Units to be produced	**7,500**
Goods available for sale..	12,000
Desired ending inventory of finished goods (50% of August's sales) ...	(3,000)
Quantity of goods sold	9,000

7,500 * 3 pounds * 40% = **9,000**

(d) "Units to be produced" each month (see answer to part *c*) * 3 pounds per unit.

Note: In the total column, the beginning and ending inventory figures represent the number of pounds on hand at April 1, 2002 and June 30, 2002, respectively. Thus, the "raw materials available for use" line does not add across.

e. | *Cash payments for:* | *April* | *May* | *June* | *Total* |
|---|---:|---:|---:|---:|
| March purchases .... | $ 26,280[e] | | | $ 26,280 |
| April purchases .... | 125,280 | $ 31,320 | | 156,600 |
| May purchases .... | | 126,720 | $ 31,680 | 158,400 |
| June purchases .... | | | 116,640 | 116,640 |
| Total cash payments .... | $151,560 | $158,040 | $148,320 | $457,920 |

(e) Purchases from February and all prior months would have been fully paid by the end of March. Thus, the $26,280 of expected accounts payable at March 31, 2002, represents the 20% of March purchases that will be paid for in April.

Note: Each month's "purchases of raw materials" in pounds (see answer to part *d*) is multiplied by $6.00 to determine the dollar amount of raw material purchases, which is then multiplied by 80% in the month of purchase and 20% in the following month to determine cash payments.

E15-1.

a. The president's remark ignores the misleading result of arbitrarily allocated fixed expenses.

b.
Current net income of company		$10,000
Less: Lost contribution margin of Division B		(10,000)
Add: Division B direct fixed expenses that would be eliminated:		
Total Division B fixed expenses per report	$11,000	
Less: Allocated corporate ($21,000 / 3 divisions)	(7,000)	4,000
Company net income without Division B.......................		**$ 4,000**

c. Never arbitrarily allocate fixed expenses!

E15-3.

a. Cost formula = $19,400 + $7.70 per machine hour
Budget = $19,400 + ($7.70 * 6,700 machine hours) = **$70,990**

b.
	Original Budget (6,700 MH)	Flexed Budget (7,060 MH)	Actual Cost	Variance
Total maintenance cost.	$70,990	$73,762 #	$68,940	**$4,822** F

  # Flexed budget = $19,400 + ($7.70 * 7,060 machine hours) = $73,762

E15-5.

a. Standard hours allowed = 3.5 hours * 24 tune-ups = 84 hours
Efficiency variance was 6 hours unfavorable, therefore actual hours
= 84 + 6 = **90 hours.**

Standard labor cost allowed for actual hours ($15 per hour * 90 hours) ...	$1,350
Less: Favorable labor rate variance	(81)
Actual total labor cost...	**$1,269**

Actual labor rate per hour = $1,269 / 90 hours = **$14.10 per hour**

b. Direct labor efficiency variance:
(Standard hours – Actual hours) * Standard rate
(84 – 90) * $15 = **$90 U**

c. Less skilled, lower paid workers took longer than standard to get the work done. Net variance is $9 U ($90 U – $81 F). This was not a good trade-off based on the variance. From a qualitative viewpoint, less skilled workers may not do as good of a job.

E15-7.

a. Purchase price variance = (Standard price – Actual price) * Actual quantity purchased
    = ($8.00 per board foot – **???** actual price) * 19,000 board feet purchased = $2,850 U.
    Thus, the purchase price per board foot was $0.15 U ($2,850 U / 19,000), or **$8.15.**

b. 1,500 units produced * 12 board feet per unit = **18,000 standard board feet allowed.**

c. Direct material usage variance = (Standard usage – Actual usage) * Standard price =
    (18,000 board feet allowed – 17,200 issued into production) * $8.00 per board foot =
    $6,400 F

d. The purchasing manager may have purchased higher-than-standard *quality* raw
    material inputs. This may have allowed Dutko, Inc., to reduce waste and spoilage,
    resulting in a favorable raw materials usage variance that more than offset the $0.15
    per board foot unfavorable price variance.   Based on the variances during November,
    this is a good trade-off for the management of Dutko, Inc., to make.

E15-9.

	Original Budget	*Flexed Budget*	*Actual*	*Variance*
a. Direct labor	$1,800	$1,716 #	$1,888	$172 U

2,860 books / 20 books per hour = 143 standard hours allowed * $ 12 per hour
= $1,716 flexed budget.

b. Direct labor efficiency variance = (143 standard hours – 160 actual hours)
    = **17 hours U.**

c. Direct labor rate variance = (Standard rate – Actual rate) * Actual hours
    = ($12 – ($1,888 / 160 hours)) * 160 hours = ($12 – $11.80) * 160 = **$32 F**

E15-11.

a. *Raw material purchase price variance:*
    (Standard price – Actual price) * Actual quantity purchased
    ($5.00 – $4.95) * 7,400 pounds = **$370 F**

b. *Raw material usage variance:*
    (Standard usage – Actual usage) * Standard price
    ((2,000 cases * 4 pounds) – 8,300 pounds) * $5.00 per pound = **$1,500 U**

c. *Direct labor rate variance:*
    (Standard rate – Actual rate) * Actual hours
    ($13.00 – $13.50 #) * 5,800 hours = **$2,900 U**
     # Actual rate: $78,300 / 5,800 hours = $13.50

E15-11. *(continued)*

   d. **Direct labor efficiency variance:**
     (Standard hours – Actual hours) * Standard rate
     ((2,000 cases * 3 hours) – 5,800) * $13.00 = **$2,600 F**

   e. **Variable overhead spending variance:**
     (Standard rate – Actual rate) * Actual hours
     ($6.00 – $6.15 #) * 5,800 hours = **$870 U**
     # Actual rate: $35,670 / 5,800 hours = $6.15

   f. **Variable overhead efficiency variance:**
     (Standard hours – Actual hours) * Standard rate
     ((2,000 cases * 3 hours) – 5,800) * $6.00 = **$1,200 F**

   Explanation of results: In order to create a favorable purchase price variance, the purchasing manager may have purchased lower-than-standard *quality* raw material inputs. This may have caused an excess amount of waste and spoilage, resulting in an unfavorable raw materials usage variance that *by far* exceeded the cost savings of $0.05 per pound. The unfavorable labor rate variance of $0.50 per hour may have been caused by using a more skilled and/or experienced workforce than was anticipated. However, this cost was largely offset by increased labor efficiency (i.e., less down-time, re-work). The favorable labor efficiency variance caused a favorable variable overhead efficiency variance because variable overhead is applied on the basis of direct labor hours.

P15-13.

	Simple	*Complex*
a. Work hours per day	7.5	7.5
Divided by: Standard processing time per claim (in hours) ...	0.75	2.5
Standard number of claims processed (per day per worker)...	10.0	3.0
Multiplied by: Number of days in the month	20.0	20.0
Standard claims processed (per month per worker)	200.0	60.0
Claims processed	3,000	600
Standard number of workers required for the month	**15**	**10**

Thus, a total of **25** workers should have been available to process the April claims.

b. Actual number of workers	27
Standard number of workers required for the month	25
Efficiency variance, in number of workers	**2 U**
Efficiency variance, in dollars (2 workers * $ 90 per day * 20 days) ...	**$3,600 U**

P15-15.

a. Predetermined overhead application rate:

$$= \frac{\text{Estimated Overhead \$}}{\text{Estimated Activity}} = \frac{\$36,000}{(40,000 \text{ units} * 0.5 \text{ hours})} = \textbf{\$1.80 per machine hour}$$

b. 39,000 units produced * 0.5 machine hours per unit = **19,500 machine hours allowed.**

c. Applied overhead = $1.80 * 19,500 hours = **$35,100**

d. ($37,000 actual overhead incurred – $35,100 overhead applied)
= **$1,900 underapplied.**

e. ($36,000 budgeted overhead – $37,000 actual overhead) = **$1,000 U budget variance.**

((20,000 budgeted hours – 19,500 standard hours allowed for units produced) * $1.80 predetermined overhead application rate) = **$900 U volume variance.**

Cost Analysis for Decision Making

E16-1.

    a. *Differential cost:* What costs will differ if a friend comes along?

    b. *Allocated cost:* How to allocate? Based on number of people, weight, number of suitcases, or what?

    c. *Sunk cost:* What costs have already been incurred and cannot be recovered, even if you don't make the trip?

    d. *Opportunity cost:* What are other opportunities for you to earn revenue? What is the cost of alternative travel for your classmate?

E16-3.

    a.

Raw materials per unit	$1.50
Direct labor per unit	1.50
Variable overhead per unit..	2.00
Fixed overhead per unit	2.00 #
Total cost per unit	$7.00

    # The fixed overhead per unit is based on the total fixed overhead for the year of $100,000 divided by the current output of 50,000 units per year.

    b. The above calculation includes an inappropriate unitization of fixed expenses. Unless the additional production of 30,000 units results in a movement to a new relevant range, total fixed expenses will not change.

    c. The offer should be accepted because it would generate a contribution margin of $1 per unit (revenue of $6 per unit less variable cost of $5 per unit).

E16-5.

    a.

```
    0——— 1——— 2——— 3——— 4
                          $65,000
                          0.6355  (Table 6-2, 4 period row,
                          ——————          12% column)
 $41,307.50 ◄──────────────────
```

    b. This is a future value problem, the opposite of present value. As shown in the diagram, $41,307.50 invested today at 12% interest compounded annually would grow to $65,000 in four years.

    c. Less could be invested today because at a higher interest rate, more interest would be earned. This can be seen by calculating the present value of $65,000 in four years at an interest rate greater than 12%. As can be seen in Table 6-2, the present value factors are smaller as interest rates get higher.

E16-7.

a. If the investment is too high, the net present value will be too low.

b. If the cost of capital is too low, the net present value will be too high.

c. If the cash flows from the project are too high, the net present value will be too high.

d. If the number of years over which the project will generate cash flows is too low, the net present value will be too low.

E16-9.

a.

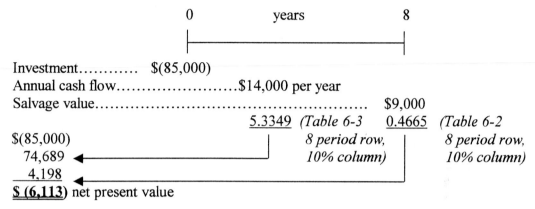

	0	years	8

Investment............ $(85,000)

Annual cash flow.......................$14,000 per year

Salvage value.. $9,000

	5.3349 *(Table 6-3*	0.4665 *(Table 6-2*
$(85,000)	*8 period row,*	*8 period row,*
74,689	*10% column)*	*10% column)*
4,198		

$ (6,113) net present value

b. Because the net present value is negative, the internal rate of return on this project will be lower than the cost of capital of 10%.

E16-11.

a. The net present value is positive $2,220 (present value of inflows of $26,220 less the investment of $24,000). Therefore, the return on investment is greater than 20%.

b. The payback period should not carry much weight at all, because it does not recognize the time value of money.

P16-13.

a. Relevant costs for the special sales order include the following:

	Per Gallon
Raw materials	$3.00
Direct labor	1.50
Variable overhead..	1.00
Distribution	1.50
Total relevant costs per gallon	$7.00

b.

	Per Gallon
Sales price	$8.00
Less: relevant costs	7.00
Contribution margin per gallon...........................	$ 1.00
Daily sales in gallons......................................	200
Daily increase in operating income	$200.00

P16-13. *(continued)*

c. Since Delmar is now operating at full capacity, relevant costs for the special sales order would include any forgone contribution margin (opportunity cost) on regular sales given up by Delmar to fulfill the special sales order:

	Per Gallon
Current sales	$10.00
Less variable costs:	
Raw materials	3.00
Direct labor...	1.50
Variable overhead	1.00
Distribution (on current sales)........................	1.00 6.50
Current contribution margin	$ 3.50

	Per Gallon
Current contribution margin	$ 3.50
Contribution margin from special order	1.00
Decrease in contribution margin	$ 2.50
Daily sales in gallons....................................	200
Daily decrease in operating income	$ 500.00

d. When Delmar is operating under conditions of idle capacity, the only relevant costs incurred in producing the gallons of root beer needed to fulfill the special order are the incremental variable costs - Delmar would not be giving up any of their current sales. Conversely, when Delmar is producing and selling root at full capacity there is no reason to accept any offer for an amount less than the current selling price and thereby accepting less contribution than is currently being earned

P16-15.

a.

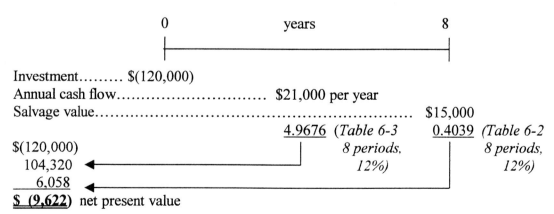

    0   years   8

Investment......... $(120,000)
Annual cash flow............................. $21,000 per year
Salvage value.. $15,000
                           4.9676 *(Table 6-3*   0.4039 *(Table 6-2*
$(120,000)   *8 periods,*   *8 periods,*
  104,320   *12%)*   *12%)*
    6,058
$ (9,622) net present value

b. Profitability index = ($110,378 present value of inflows / $120,000 investment) = **0.92**

c. Internal rate of return (actual rate of return) is considerably less than the cost of capital of 12% because the net present value is negative and the profitability index is quite low.

P16-15. *(continued)*

d. Payback period = **5.7 years**.

Investment	$(120,000)
Total return in years 1-5 ($21,000 annual cash flow * 5 years)	105,000
Return required in year 6 ($15,000 / $21,000 = 0.7 years)................	15,000
Total return in 5.7 years	$ 120,000

P16-17.

a.

Proposal	Investment	Net PV	PV of Inflows (Investment + Net PV)	Profitability Index (PV of Inflows / Outflows)
1	$50,000	$30,000	$80,000	$80,000 / $50,000 = **1.6**
2	60,000	24,000	84,000	84,000 / 60,000 = **1.4**
3	30,000	15,000	45,000	45,000 / 30,000 = **1.5**
4	45,000	9,000	54,000	54,000 / 45,000 = **1.2**

Proposal 1 is most desirable because its profitability index is the highest.

P16-19.

a. Accounting rate of return =

$$\frac{\text{Net Income}}{\text{Average Investment}} = \frac{\$29,000 - \$10,000\,\#}{(\$100,000 + \$90,000\,\#\#)\,/\,2} = \mathbf{20\%}$$

\# Depreciation expense = (Cost – Salvage) / Life
= ($80,000 – $50,000) / 3 = $10,000

\#\# Investment at end of the year = Investment at beginning of the year, less
Accumulated depreciation = $100,000 – $10,000 = $90,000

b.

Investment:		Year 1	Year 2	Year 3	Year 4
Machine	$(80,000)				
Working Capital	(20,000)				
Cash returns:					
Operations		$14,000	$24,000	$29,000	$20,000
Salvage					50,000
Working Capital					20,000
Totals	$(100,000)	$14,000	$24,000	$29,000	$90,000
PV Factor for 18%		0.8475	0.7182	0.6086	0.5158
Present value		$11,865	$17,237	$17,649	$46,422
Sum of present values	93,173				
Net present value	$ (6,827)				

Based on this analysis, the investment would *not* be made because the net present value is negative, indicating that the ROI on the project is less than the discount rate of 18%.

P16-19. *(continued)*

    c.   The net present value analytical approach is the best technique to use because it recognizes the time value of money.

CHAPTER 1

ACCOUNTING - PRESENT AND PAST

McGraw-Hill/Irwin ©The McGraw-Hill Companies, Inc., 2002

Learning Objectives

1. What is the FASB?
2. Who uses accounting information and why?
3. What is accounting?
4. What do accountants do?
5. Where did accounting come from?

McGraw-Hill/Irwin ©The McGraw-Hill Companies, Inc., 2002

Learning Objectives

6. Where did accounting standards come from?
7. What are the accounting ethical standards?
8. What is the Conceptual Framework?
9. Why do businesses report financial information?

McGraw-Hill/Irwin ©The McGraw-Hill Companies, Inc., 2002

Learning Objective 1

- What is accounting?

Accounting is the process of:

| Identifying | } | Economic information about an entity | > | For decisions and informed judgments |
| Measuring |
| Communicating |

Learning Objective 2

- Who uses accounting information and why?

Users of Accounting Information

- **Management** - planning, directing, controlling
- **Investors** - return
- **Creditors** - probability of collection
- **Employees** - job prospects and retirement benefits
- **SEC** - full disclosure of financial information

McGraw-Hill/Irwin   ©The McGraw-Hill Companies, Inc., 2002

Learning Objective 3

- What do accountants do?

McGraw-Hill/Irwin   ©The McGraw-Hill Companies, Inc., 2002

Professional Services Provided by Accountants

- Financial Accounting
- Managerial/Cost Accounting
- Auditing - Public Accounting
- Internal Auditing
- Governmental and Not-for-Profit Accounting
- Income Tax Accounting

McGraw-Hill/Irwin   ©The McGraw-Hill Companies, Inc., 2002

Learning Objective 4

- Where did accounting come from?

Early History of Accounting

- Found accounting records on Mesopotamian clay tablets from 3000 BC

- Luca Pacioli published a description of double-entry bookkeeping systems in 1494

- Industrial revolution led to non-owner managers who needed to report financial information to owners

Accounting Profession in the United States

- The Securities Act of 1933 and the Securities Exchange Act of 1934 gave the SEC the authority to establish accounting principles for SEC firms

- The SEC delegated standard setting to other organizations
  - Committee on Accounting Procedure 1939 - 1959
  - Accounting Principles Board 1959 -1973
  - Financial Accounting Standards Board 1973 - present

Learning Objective 5

- What is the FASB?

McGrawHill/Irwin   ©The McGraw-Hill Companies, Inc., 2002

Financial Accounting Standards Board

- Has issued seven concept statements
- Has issued over 140 standards statements
- Uses due process is setting standards

McGrawHill/Irwin   ©The McGraw-Hill Companies, Inc., 2002

Learning Objective 6

- Where did accounting standards come from?

McGrawHill/Irwin   ©The McGraw-Hill Companies, Inc., 2002

Other Accounting Standards

- **Cost Accounting Standards Board -** government contracts, colleges and universities that receive federal research funds

- **Governmental Accounting Standards Board** - state and local governments

- **International Accounting Standards Committee** - seeks comparability of financial statements across nations

McGrawHill/Irwin   ©The McGraw-Hill Companies, Inc., 2002

Learning Objective 7

- What are the accounting ethical standards?

McGrawHill/Irwin   ©The McGraw-Hill Companies, Inc., 2002

Ethics in the Accounting Profession

- American Institute of Certified Public Accountants
- Institute of Management Accountants

- **Integrity** - honest and forthright
- **Objectivity** - impartial and free from conflicts of interest

McGrawHill/Irwin   ©The McGraw-Hill Companies, Inc., 2002

Learning Objective 8

- What is the Conceptual Framework?

McGrawHillIrwin — ©The McGraw-Hill Companies, Inc., 2002

Conceptual Framework

- Standards are based on a foundation provided by the Statements of Financial Accounting Concepts:
  - Objectives of financial reporting
  - Qualitative characteristics of accounting information
  - Elements of financial statements
  - Recognition and measurement in financial statements
  - Using cash flow information

McGrawHillIrwin — ©The McGraw-Hill Companies, Inc., 2002

Learning Objective 9

- Why do businesses report financial information?

McGrawHillIrwin — ©The McGraw-Hill Companies, Inc., 2002

Concepts Statement No. 1: Objectives of Financial Reporting

- Intended for investors and creditors

- For assessing the amounts, timing, and uncertainty of prospective cash flows

- For providing information about economic resources and claims to those resources

McGrawHill/Irwin   ©The McGraw-Hill Companies, Inc., 2002

_____

_____

_____

_____

_____

_____

_____

CHAPTER 2

FINANCIAL STATEMENTS AND ACCOUNTING CONCEPTS/PRINCIPLES

McGraw-Hill/Irwin   ©The McGraw-Hill Companies, Inc., 2002

Learning Objectives

1. What are generally accepted accounting principle?
2. What kind of information is reported on each financial statement and how are the financial statements related?
3. What are transactions? What is the meaning and usefulness of the accounting equation?
4. What are meanings of the captions in the financial statements?

McGraw-Hill/Irwin   ©The McGraw-Hill Companies, Inc., 2002

Learning Objectives

5. Why is cash flow important?
6. What are the limitations of financial statements?
7. What is an annual report and why is it issued?
8. What are some of the business practices related to organizations?

McGraw-Hill/Irwin   ©The McGraw-Hill Companies, Inc., 2002

Learning Objective 1

- What kind of information is reported on each financial statement and how are the financial statements related?

Financial Statements

- Result of a process that begins with an economic event

- The event becomes a recorded transaction

- The transaction becomes part of a firm's financial statements

The Financial Statements

- **Balance Sheet** – financial position at the end of the period

- **Income Statement** – earnings for the period

- **Statement of Changes in Owners' Equity** – investments by and distributions to owners during the period

- **Statement of Cash Flows** – cash flows for the period

Process

Transactions → | Procedures for sorting, classifying, and presenting (**bookkeeping**)

Selection of alternative methods of reflecting the effects of certain transactions (**accounting**) | → | Financial statements |

McGrawHillIrwin   ©The McGraw-Hill Companies, Inc., 2002

Learning Objective 2

- What are transactions? What is the meaning and usefulness of the accounting equation?

McGrawHillIrwin   ©The McGraw-Hill Companies, Inc., 2002

Transactions

- Economic interchanges between entities
- Examples are:
  - A sale
  - A purchase
  - Receipts of cash by borrower
  - Payment of cash by lender

McGrawHillIrwin   ©The McGraw-Hill Companies, Inc., 2002

Balance Sheet

- Financial position at the end of a period - A snapshot at a point in time
- Also called Statement of Financial Position
- Contains three parts:
  - Assets
  - Liabilities
  - Owners' Equity
- **Assets = Liabilities + Owners' Equity**

Learning Objective 3

- What are the meanings of the captions in the financial statements?

Assets

- Probable future economic benefits
- Resources owned
- Can be classified as current or long-term

Examples of Assets

- **Cash** – cash on hand or in banks
- **Accounts Receivable** – amounts due from customers
- **Merchandise Inventory** – merchandise acquired but not yet sold
- **Equipment** – assets used in the business
- Less: **Accumulated Depreciation** – cost of equipment estimated to have been used up

McGrawHillIrwin   ©The McGrawHill Companies, Inc., 2002

Liabilities

- Probable future sacrifices of economic benefits
- Obligations
- Can be classified as current or long-term

McGrawHillIrwin   ©The McGrawHill Companies, Inc., 2002

Examples of Liabilities

- **Accounts Payable** - amounts owed to suppliers of merchandise inventory
- **Long-term Debt** – amounts borrowed but will not be repaid within one year

McGrawHillIrwin   ©The McGrawHill Companies, Inc., 2002

Income Statement

- Summary of the earnings for a period
- Consists of:
  - **Revenues**
  - **Expenses**

- Covers a period of time

- Also called Statement of Earnings, or Profit and Loss Statement, or Statement of Operations

---

Income Statement Sections

- **Revenues** - operating activities for the period - often reported as Net Sales

- **Expenses** - Costs incurred in generating revenues

Examples of Expenses

- **Cost of Goods Sold** – total cost of inventory delivered to customers as a result of sales
- **Selling, General, and Administrative Expenses** – operating expenses of an entity
- **Interest Expense** – cost of using borrowed funds
- **Income Taxes**

More Income Statement Sections

- **Gross Profit** – difference between sales and cost of goods sold

- **Income From Operations** – an important measure of a firm's activities

- **Income Before Taxes** – income from operations less interest expense

---

More Income Statement Sections

- **Net Income** – income remaining after all expenses have been deducted

- **Net Income Per Share of Common Stock Outstanding** – used in measuring the market value of a share of common stock

---

Statement of Changes in Owners' Equity

- Also called Statement of Changes in Capital Stock, or Statement of Changes in Retained Earnings

- Explains the changes that occurred in the components of owners' equity during the year

Owners' Equity

- Paid-In Capital
  - **Common Stock** - at par value
  - **Additional Paid-In Capital** – difference between total amount invested by the owners and the par or stated value of the stock
- **Retained Earnings** – cumulative net income retained in the business
  - **Dividends** – distribution of earnings to owners

Learning Objective 5

- Why is cash flow important?

Statement of Cash Flows

- Sources and uses of cash
- Covers a period of time
- Includes:
  - Operating Activities
  - Investing Activities
  - Financing Activities

Cash Flows from Operating Activities

- Start with Net Income
- Add back Depreciation Expense
- Deduct (add) increases (decreases) in current assets
- Deduct (add) decreases (increases) in current liabilities

McGraw-Hill/Irwin   ©The McGraw-Hill Companies, Inc., 2002

Cash Flows from Investing Activities

- Cash used to purchase long-lived assets
- Cash received from sales of long-lived assets
- Other changes in cash investments

McGraw-Hill/Irwin   ©The McGraw-Hill Companies, Inc., 2002

Cash Flows from Financing Activities

- Cash raised from the sale of long-term debt and common stock
- Cash paid to reduce long-term debt and stock outstanding

McGraw-Hill/Irwin   ©The McGraw-Hill Companies, Inc., 2002

Financial Statement Relationships

- All financial statements are related

- Net Income from the Income Statement affects Retained Earnings on the Balance Sheet

- The Income Statement and the Balance Sheet affect the Statement of Cash Flows

McGraw-Hill/Irwin   ©The McGraw-Hill Companies, Inc., 2002

Learning Objective 4

- What are generally accepted accounting principles?

McGraw-Hill/Irwin   ©The McGraw-Hill Companies, Inc., 2002

Concepts and Principles

- **Accounting Entity** – entity for which financial statements are being prepared – can be a proprietorship, partnership, corporation, or group of corporations

- **Going Concern** – presumption that the entity will continue to operate in the future

- **Unit of Measurement** – in the United States, the dollar is the measurement unit for all transactions

McGraw-Hill/Irwin   ©The McGraw-Hill Companies, Inc., 2002

Concepts and Principles

- **Cost Principle** – transactions are recorded at their original cost as measured in dollars
- **Objectivity** – a given transaction should be recorded in the same way in all situations
- **Accounting Period** – the period of time selected for recording results
- **Matching** – expenses are matched with the revenues that produced them

McGraw-Hill/Irwin ©The McGraw-Hill Companies, Inc., 2002

Concepts and Principles

- **Accrual Accounting** – revenue recognized at the time of sale and expenses recognized when incurred
- **Consistency** – maintaining the method of accounting for a particular type of transaction
- **Full Disclosure** – all necessary information is presented in the financial statements and notes so investors will not be misled

McGraw-Hill/Irwin ©The McGraw-Hill Companies, Inc., 2002

Concepts and Principles

- **Materiality** – absolute exactness is not necessary as long as not misleading
- **Conservatism** – make judgments and estimates that result in lower profits and asset valuations rather than higher profits and higher asset valuations

McGraw-Hill/Irwin ©The McGraw-Hill Companies, Inc., 2002

Learning Objective 6

- What are the limitations of financial statements?

Limitations of Financial Statements

- Financial statements do not reflect qualitative economic variables

- Balance sheet does not reflect current values

- Estimates are used in many areas of accounting

More Limitations of Financial Statements

- Two firms may use different accounting methods, making comparisons difficult

- Inflation is not included in accounting procedures

- Financial statements do not reflect opportunity costs

Learning Objective 7

- What is an annual report and why is it issued?

McGraw-Hill/Irwin   ©The McGraw-Hill Companies, Inc., 2002

Annual Report

- Distributed to shareholders
- Contains:
  - Financial statements
  - External auditor's report
  - Footnotes and explanatory comments
  - Letters from the CEO and president

McGraw-Hill/Irwin   ©The McGraw-Hill Companies, Inc., 2002

Learning Objective 8

- What are some of the business practices related to organizations?

McGraw-Hill/Irwin   ©The McGraw-Hill Companies, Inc., 2002

Business Practices

- Organizing a business
  - **Sole proprietorship**
  - **Partnership**
  - **Corporation**
- **Fiscal Year** – annual reporting period
- **Par value** – arbitrary value assigned to stock; no relationship to value
- **Parent and subsidiary corporations** – parent owns at least a majority of the stock of another corporation

McGraw-Hill/Irwin   ©The McGraw-Hill Companies, Inc., 2002

_____

_____

_____

_____

_____

_____

_____

CHAPTER 3

FUNDAMENTAL
INTERPRETATIONS
MADE FROM
FINANCIAL
STATEMENT DATA

McGraw-Hill/Irwin   ©The McGraw-Hill Companies, Inc., 2002

Learning Objectives

1. Why are financial statement ratios important?
2. How is return on investment calculated and why is it important?
3. What is the DuPont model and what do margin and turnover mean?
4. What is the significance of return on equity and how is it calculated?

McGraw-Hill/Irwin   ©The McGraw-Hill Companies, Inc., 2002

Learning Objectives

5. What does liquidity mean and why is it important?
6. How are working capital, current ratio, and acid-test ratio calculated and why are they significant?
7. How can trend analysis be used most effectively?

McGraw-Hill/Irwin   ©The McGraw-Hill Companies, Inc., 2002

Learning Objective 1

- Why are financial statement ratios important?

McGrawHillIrwin ©The McGrawHill Companies, Inc., 2002

Financial Ratios and Trend Analysis

- A ratio is the relationship between two numbers
- Ratios are useful for comparing different sized firms
- Average ratios for an industry are useful for comparisons
- A trend is comparing ratios over several time periods
- Trend analysis provides are more meaningful comparisons

McGrawHillIrwin ©The McGrawHill Companies, Inc., 2002

Learning Objective 2

- How is return on investment calculated and why is it important?

McGrawHillIrwin ©The McGrawHill Companies, Inc., 2002

Return on Investment Calculations

- Rate of return =
  Amount of return / Amount of investment
- Return on investment is a measure of profitability
- Derived from the interest calculation of:
  Interest = Principal x Rate x Time

McGrawHill/Irwin   ©The McGraw-Hill Companies, Inc., 2002

_____

_____

_____

_____

_____

_____

_____

Return on Investment and Risk

- In evaluating investments, risk must also be considered
- Risk relates to the range of outcomes from an activity; wider range = greater risk
- In general, higher risk = higher return

McGrawHill/Irwin   ©The McGraw-Hill Companies, Inc., 2002

_____

_____

_____

_____

_____

_____

_____

Financial Statements and Return on Investment

- Also called Return on Assets
- The amount of return = Net Income
- The amount of the investment = Average Total Assets
- Describes the rate of return management was able to earn on the assets available to use during the year
- May also be calculated as Operating Income / Average Operating Assets

McGrawHill/Irwin   ©The McGraw-Hill Companies, Inc., 2002

_____

_____

_____

_____

_____

_____

_____

Learning Objective 3

- What is the DuPont model and what do margin and turnover mean?

The DuPont Model

- An expansion of the basic return on investment calculation

- Return on Investment =

$$\frac{\text{Net Income}}{\text{Sales}} \times \frac{\text{Sales}}{\text{Average Total Assets}}$$

- Net Income / Sales = Margin

- Sales / Average Total Assets = Asset Turnover

Margin and Asset Turnover

- Margin indicates that some sales revenues must result in net income if the firm is to be profitable

- Turnover indicates how efficiently the firm is using its assets to generate revenue

Learning Objective 4

What is the significance of return on equity and how is it calculated?

McGrawHillIrwin ©The McGraw-Hill Companies, Inc., 2002

Return on Equity

- Return on Equity is a special case application of the rate of return concept

- Return on Equity =

Net Income
Average Owners' Equity

McGrawHillIrwin ©The McGraw-Hill Companies, Inc., 2002

Learning Objective 5

- What does liquidity mean and why is it important?

McGrawHillIrwin ©The McGraw-Hill Companies, Inc., 2002

Working Capital and Measures of Liquidity

- Liquidity is the firm's ability to meet its current obligations

- Working capital is the excess of a firm's current assets over its current liabilities

  - Current assets are cash and other assets likely to be converted to cash within a year

  - Current liabilities are those obligations expected to be paid within a year

Measures of Liquidity

- Working Capital =
  Current Assets less Current Liabilities

- Current Ratio =
  Current Assets divided by Current Liabilities

- Acid-Test Ratio =
  Cash and Accounts Receivable divided by Current Liabilities

Learning Objective 6

- How are working capital, current ratio, and acid-test ratio calculated and why are they significant?

Current Ratio

- The trend in the current ratio is the most useful in judging a firm's current bill-paying ability

- As a general rule, a current ratio of 2.0 is considered adequate

- The higher the current ratio, the better – up to a point

McGrawHill/Irwin   ©The McGrawHill Companies, Inc., 2002

Acid-Test Ratio

- Also known as the **Quick Ratio**

- The Acid-Test Ratio is a more conservative measure of liquidity since inventory is not included in its calculation

- As a general rule, an Acid-Test Ratio of 1.0 is considered adequate

McGrawHill/Irwin   ©The McGrawHill Companies, Inc., 2002

Learning Objective 7

- How can trend analysis be used most effectively?

McGrawHill/Irwin   ©The McGrawHill Companies, Inc., 2002

Trend Analysis

- Graph return against the year, with the years listed on the horizontal axis

- The more compressed the graph, the more pronounced the peaks and valleys

- See following graph of margin and turnover for Intel Corporation

---

Intel Corporation Margin and Turnover, 1995 - 1999

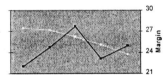

CHAPTER 4

THE BOOKKEEPING PROCESS AND TRANSACTION ANALYSIS

McGraw-Hill/Irwin   ©The McGraw-Hill Companies, Inc., 2002

Learning Objectives

1. How can the basic accounting equation be expanded to include revenues and expenses?
2. How does the expanded accounting equation stay in balance after every transaction?
3. How is the income statement linked to the balance sheet through owners' equity?
4. What are the meanings of the terms journal, ledger, T-account, account balance, debit, credit, and closing the books?

McGraw-Hill/Irwin   ©The McGraw-Hill Companies, Inc., 2002

Learning Objectives

5. How is the bookkeeping system a mechanical adaptation of the expanded accounting equation?
6. How is a transaction analyzed, how is a journal entry prepared, and how is the effect of a transaction on working capital determined?
7. What are the five questions of transaction analysis?

McGraw-Hill/Irwin   ©The McGraw-Hill Companies, Inc., 2002

Learning Objective 1

- How can the basic accounting equation be expanded to include revenues and expenses?

McGrawHillIrwin   ©The McGrawHill Companies, Inc., 2002

Bookkeeping/Accounting Process

- The process begins with transactions

- The transactions are reflected in the financial statements

- One must know the mechanical process to understand the effects of transactions on the financial statements

McGrawHillIrwin   ©The McGrawHill Companies, Inc., 2002

The Balance Sheet Equations

- The basic equation is:
  Assets = Liabilities + Owners' Equity
- Since Owners' Equity consists of Paid-In Capital and Retained Earnings, the equation can be restated as:
- **Assets = Liabilities + (Paid-In Capital + Retained Earnings)**

McGrawHillIrwin   ©The McGrawHill Companies, Inc., 2002

The Balance Sheet Equations

- Since Retained Earnings is computed as Beginning Retained Earnings plus Revenues and less Expenses, the basic equation can be restated as:

Assets = Liabilities + (Paid-In Capital + Beginning Retained Earnings + Revenues – Expenses)

McGrawHillIrwin · ©The McGraw-Hill Companies, Inc., 2002

Learning Objective 2

- How does the expanded accounting equation stay in balance after every transaction?

McGrawHillIrwin · ©The McGraw-Hill Companies, Inc., 2002

EXHIBIT 4-1
Transaction Summary

| | | ASSETS | | | LIABILITIES | | | OWNERS' EQUITY | | |
Transaction	Cash	Accounts Receivable	Merchandise Inventory	Equipment	Notes Payable	Accounts Payable	Paid-In Capital	Retained Earnings	Revenue	Expenses
1.	+30						+30			
2.	-25			+25						
3.	+15				+15					
4.	-10		+20			+10				
5.	+2	+5		-7						
6.	+5	-5								
Total	17	0	20	18	15	10	30			
7.	Revenues	+20							+20	
7.	Expenses	20	-12							-12
8.						+3				-3
Total	17	20	8	18	15	13	30		+20	-15

+5 ◄ ─────

McGrawHillIrwin · ©The McGraw-Hill Companies, Inc., 2002

Learning Objective 3

- How is the income statement linked to the balance sheet through owners' equity?

McGraw-Hill/Irwin ©The McGraw-Hill Companies, Inc., 2002

Linking the Income Statement and the Balance Sheet

- The Net Income on the Income Statement gets into the Balance Sheet through the Retained Earnings section of Owners' Equity

- See the previous slide for an example

McGraw-Hill/Irwin ©The McGraw-Hill Companies, Inc., 2002

Learning Objective 4

- What are the meanings of the terms journal, ledger, T-account, account balance, debit, credit, and closing the books?

McGraw-Hill/Irwin ©The McGraw-Hill Companies, Inc., 2002

Bookkeeping Jargon and Procedures

- **Journal** – where transactions are initially recorded
- **Post** – to record
- **Ledger** – a set of accounts for each category of asset, liability, and owners' equity
- **Chart of accounts** – an index to the ledger
- **T-Account** – an account format that looks like a "T." One side indicates an addition; the other a subtraction from the account
- **Debit** – the left side
- **Credit** – the right side

Learning Objective 5

- How is the bookkeeping system a mechanical adaptation of the expanded accounting equation?

The Bookkeeping System

- Debits must always equal credits
- Asset accounts will normally have debit balances
- Increases in assets are entered as debits; decreases are entered as credits
- Liabilities and Owners' Equity are the opposite of Assets. Debits are decreases and credits are increases

Journal Entries

- The journal is the book of original entry
- The format for a journal entry is as follows:

Date   Dr.   Account name   Amount
        Cr.   Account name   Amount

- Note the date is entered for reference
- Dr. and Cr. are used for debit and credit
- A journal entry may have more than one debit and more than one credit

McGrawHillIrwin   ©The McGrawHill Companies, Inc., 2002

Learning Objective 6

- How is a transaction analyzed, how is a journal entry prepared, and how is the effect of a transaction on the financial statements determined?

McGrawHillIrwin   ©The McGrawHill Companies, Inc., 2002

Transaction Effects - Balance Sheet

- The horizontal model is an alternative to using T-accounts and journal entries
- The model is as follows:

Balance Sheet   **Income Statement**

Assets = Liabilities + Owners' Equity ← Net Income = Revenues − Expenses

(Accounts and amounts affected by transactions are entered under the appropriate categories)

McGrawHillIrwin   ©The McGrawHill Companies, Inc., 2002

Adjusting Entries

- Made to reflect accrual accounting in the financial statements

- Results in revenues and expenses being reported in the appropriate fiscal period

- Two types of adjusting entries
  - Accruals
  - Reclassifications

McGrawHillIrwin ©The McGrawHill Companies, Inc., 2002

Accruals and Reclassifications

- **Accruals** - transactions for which cash has not yet been received or paid, but revenues and expenses need to be matched

- **Reclassifications** – the initial recording of a transaction must be reclassified to reflect when revenues were earned or when expenses were incurred

McGrawHillIrwin ©The McGrawHill Companies, Inc., 2002

Accruals

- Example: Work performed by employees in March, but paid in April

- At the end of March debit Wages Expense and credit Wages Payable

- Example: Interest earned in March, but not received

- At the end of March debit Interest Receivable and credit Interest Revenue

McGrawHillIrwin ©The McGrawHill Companies, Inc., 2002

Reclassifications

- Example: Supplies are purchased in February and are recorded as an asset. Then the supplies are used.

- The expense Supplies Expense should be debited and the asset Supplies should be credited for the amount of supplies used

- If the purchased supplies were debited to Supplies Expense when purchased, the unused supplies should be debited to the asset account and the Supplies Expense account should be credited

McGrawHillIrwin   ©The McGraw-Hill Companies, Inc., 2002

Adjusting Entries Revisited

- Generally, every adjusting entry affects both the Balance Sheet and the Income Statement

- After the adjusting entries have been made, the account balances are determined, and the financial statements are prepared

McGrawHillIrwin   ©The McGraw-Hill Companies, Inc., 2002

Learning Objective 7

- What are the five questions of transaction analysis?

McGrawHillIrwin   ©The McGraw-Hill Companies, Inc., 2002

Five Transaction Analysis Questions

- What's going on?
- What accounts are affected?
- How are they affected?
- Does the Balance Sheet balance? (Do the debits equal the credits?)
- Does my analysis make sense?

McGrawHill/Irwin · ©The McGraw-Hill Companies, Inc., 2002

What's Going On?

- To analyze a transaction, the transaction must be understood
- It is necessary to understand the entity for which accounting is being done and standard business practices

McGrawHill/Irwin · ©The McGraw-Hill Companies, Inc., 2002

What Accounts Are Affected?

- Often the accounts affected are explained by understanding what is going on
- Can also be answered by the process of elimination

McGrawHill/Irwin · ©The McGraw-Hill Companies, Inc., 2002

How Are They Affected?

- Answer this by using "increasing" or "decreasing"
- Then relate the increases and decreases to debits and credits to the appropriate accounts
- If using the horizontal model, debits and credits are avoided

McGraw-Hill/Irwin ©The McGraw-Hill Companies, Inc., 2002

Does the Balance Sheet Balance?

- If using the horizontal model, the answer is found easily
- Remember that debits must equal credits and assets must equal liabilities plus owners' equity

McGraw-Hill/Irwin ©The McGraw-Hill Companies, Inc., 2002

Does My Analysis Make Sense?

- Think about the effect of the transaction on the financial statements
- Do the effects that you have recorded reflect what happened?

McGraw-Hill/Irwin ©The McGraw-Hill Companies, Inc., 2002

CHAPTER 5

ACCOUNTING FOR AND PRESENTATION OF CURRENT ASSETS

McGraw-Hill/Irwin   ©The McGraw-Hill Companies, Inc., 2002

Learning Objectives

1. What is included in the cash amount reported on the balance sheet?

2. What are the features of an internal control system, and why are internal controls important?

3. What is the bank reconciliation procedure?

4. How are short-term marketable securities reported on the balance sheet?

McGraw-Hill/Irwin   ©The McGraw-Hill Companies, Inc., 2002

Learning Objectives

5. How are accounts receivable reported on the balance sheet, including the valuation allowances for estimated uncollectible accounts and estimated cash discounts?

6. How are notes receivable and related accrued interest reported on the balance sheet?

7. How are inventories reported on the balance sheet?

McGraw-Hill/Irwin   ©The McGraw-Hill Companies, Inc., 2002

Learning Objectives

8. What are the alternative inventory cost flow assumptions, and what are their respective effects on the income statement and balance sheet when price levels are changing?

9. What are the effects of inventory errors on the balance sheet and income statement?

10. What are prepaid expenses, and how are they reported on the balance sheet?

Learning Objective 1

- What is included in the cash amount reported on the balance sheet?

Cash and Cash Equivalents

- **Cash** includes money on hand in change funds, petty cash, undeposited receipts, and checking and savings accounts

- **Cash equivalents** are short-term investments easily convertible to cash

- **Cash management** is concerned with maximizing earnings by having as much cash as feasible invested for the longest possible time

Learning Objective 2

- What are the features of an internal control system, and why are internal controls important?

Internal Control System

- A process designed to provide reasonable assurance that objects are achieved with respect to:
  - The effectiveness and efficiency of the operations
  - The reliability of the organization's financial reporting
  - The organization's compliance with applicable laws and regulations
- Includes financial and administrative controls

Financial Controls

- Are related to the concept of separation of duties
- Includes a system of checks and balances such that one individual is not involved in an entire transaction
- Example: individual preparing checks does not sign the checks

Administrative Controls

- Frequently included in policy and procedures manuals

- Reflected in management reviews of operations and activities

- Example: evaluating a customer's credit history before approving a credit sale

Learning Objective 3

- What is the bank reconciliation procedure?

Bank Reconciliation

- Used to determine that the amount of cash shown in the general ledger is the same as the cash reported by the bank

- Differences may result due to:

    - Timing differences
    - Errors

Timing Differences

- **Deposits in transit** – included in firm's cash account, but not yet recorded by the bank

- **Outstanding checks** – deducted from firm's cash account, but not yet deducted by the bank

- **Bank service charges** – deducted by the bank, but not yet deducted from firm's cash account

- **NSF checks** – not sufficient funds- checks that have bounced from a customer's account

McGraw-Hill/Irwin   ©The McGraw-Hill Companies, Inc., 2002

Errors

- Can be made by either the firm or the bank

- If the error is in the recording of cash transactions on the firm's books, an adjusting entry must be made to correct it

- Often a very time-consuming process to find errors

McGraw-Hill/Irwin   ©The McGraw-Hill Companies, Inc., 2002

Bank Reconciliation Example

Bank Records		Company Books	
Indicated balance	$5,233.21	Indicated balance	$4,614.58
Add: Deposits in transit	859.10	Add: Interest earned	28.91
Less: Outstanding checks	(1,526.58)	Less: Service charge	(43.76)
Reconciled balance	$4,565.73	NSF Check	(35.00)
		Reconciled balance	$4,565.73

McGraw-Hill/Irwin   ©The McGraw-Hill Companies, Inc., 2002

Learning Objective 4

- How are short-term marketable securities reported on the balance sheet?

Short-Term Marketable Securities

- Part of a firm's cash management strategy

- Prudent use of short-term marketable securities as investments can improve ROI

- Examples: U.S. treasury securities, commercial paper, and bank certificates of deposit

Reporting of Short-Term Marketable Securities

- Short-term marketable debt securities that are classified as held-to-maturity are reported at cost

- Debt and equity securities that are classified as trading or available-for-sale securities are reported at market value

- Interest on these securities is accrued as it is earned

Learning Objective 5

- How are accounts receivable reported on the balance sheet, including the valuation allowances for estimated uncollectible accounts and estimated cash discounts?

McGrawHill/Irwin   ©The McGraw-Hill Companies, Inc., 2002

Accounts Receivable

- Are reported on the Balance Sheet at net realizable value – the amount expected to be received from customers
- The amount initially recorded may be different from net realizable due to:
  - Bad debts
  - Cash discounts

McGrawHill/Irwin   ©The McGraw-Hill Companies, Inc., 2002

Bad Debts

- Bad debts are inevitable when sales are made on credit
- Credit managers are able to estimate the amount of bad debts fairly accurately
- Two methods are used to estimate bad debts:
  - Percentage of credit sales
  - Aging of accounts receivable

McGrawHill/Irwin   ©The McGraw-Hill Companies, Inc., 2002

Percentage of Credit Sales

- An estimated percentage of credit sales losses is multiplied by the total credit sales

- An entry is made in the firm's records increasing bad debt expense and increasing a valuation adjustment account

Aging of Accounts Receivable

- Involves a detailed analysis of age of accounts receivable

- The longer an account is past due, the less likely the firm is to collect the amount owed

- An entry is made in the firm's records increasing bad debt expense and increasing a valuation adjustment account

Entries Related to Bad Debts

- Recording the estimated amount:

Bad Debt Expense	xx	
Allowance for Bad Debts		xx

- Writing off an uncollectible account:

Allowance for Bad Debts	xx	
Accounts Receivable		xx

Cash Discounts

- Are used to encourage prompt payment
- Credit terms often abbreviated as 2/10, n30, meaning a 2 percent discount may be taken if the account is paid within 10 days, and the net amount is due in 30 days
- The estimation of cash discounts is similar to the estimation of bad debts

McGrawHill/Irwin   ©The McGraw-Hill Companies, Inc., 2002

Learning Objective 6

- How are notes receivable and related accrued interest reported on the balance sheet?

McGrawHill/Irwin   ©The McGraw-Hill Companies, Inc., 2002

Notes Receivable

- A firm may convert and account receivable into a note receivable if a customer has developed difficulties paying the amount due
- A note receivable is a formal document that includes maturity date, collateral, and penalties
- Notes receivable are also used when lending funds to another entity

McGrawHill/Irwin   ©The McGraw-Hill Companies, Inc., 2002

Interest Accrual

- If interest is to be paid on a note receivable at the maturity of the note, the holder accrues interest on a monthly basis

- This shows that interest income has been earned

- Use the account Interest Receivable

Learning Objective 7

- How are inventories reported on the balance sheet?

Inventories

- For merchandising and manufacturing firms, the sale of inventory is the major, ongoing source of revenue

- Accounting for inventory is basically the same for all firms

- As inventory is sold, it is moved from an asset to an expense – Cost of Goods Sold

- Amount of cost of goods sold depends on the cost flow assumption used by the firm

Inventory Cost Flow Assumptions

- Four principal alternative cost flow assumptions:
  - Specific Identification
  - Weighted Average
  - First-in, First-out (FIFO)
  - Last-in, First-out (LIFO)
- Only cost flow assumptions, not physical flow assumptions

McGrawHillIrwin   ©The McGrawHill Companies, Inc., 2002

Learning Objective 8

- What are the alternative inventory cost flow assumptions, and what are their respective effects on the income statement and balance sheet when price levels are changing?

McGrawHillIrwin   ©The McGrawHill Companies, Inc., 2002

Specific Identification

- Links cost with the physical flow of goods

- When and item is sold, the cost of that specific item is moved to cost of goods sold

- Not practical for firms with a large number of inventory items

McGrawHillIrwin   ©The McGrawHill Companies, Inc., 2002

Weighted-Average

- Applied to individual items of inventory
- Is not a simple average of the costs of the inventory items; the average is weighted by the number of units purchased at a specific price
- The weighted average cost is then multiplied by the number of units sold to determine cost of goods sold, and by the number of units in ending inventory to determine the balance sheet valuation

McGrawHillIrwin   ©The McGrawHill Companies, Inc., 2002

First-In, First-Out (FIFO)

- The first costs in to inventory are the first costs out to cost of goods sold
- The oldest costs are transferred to cost of goods sold
- The balance sheet reports the most current costs of inventory

McGrawHillIrwin   ©The McGrawHill Companies, Inc., 2002

Last-In, First-Out (LIFO)

- The most recent costs of inventory are transferred to the income statement - cost of goods sold – when items are sold
- The oldest costs are reported on the balance sheet

McGrawHillIrwin   ©The McGrawHill Companies, Inc., 2002

Impact of Changing Costs

- In times of rising costs, LIFO results in lower ending inventory amounts and higher cost of goods sold than FIFO

- When inventory purchase costs are decreasing, FIFO results in lower ending inventory amounts and higher cost of goods sold than LIFO

McGrawHillIrwin ©The McGraw-Hill Companies, Inc., 2002

Selecting an Inventory Cost-Flow Assumption

- When rates of inflation are low, most financial managers choose FIFO

- In periods of high inflation, managers choose LIFO to avoid high taxes

- However, consistency requires the use of a single cost-flow assumption

- If a change in methods is made, the effect of the change on both the balance sheet and the income statement must be disclosed

McGrawHillIrwin ©The McGraw-Hill Companies, Inc., 2002

Inventory Accounting System Alternatives

- Accounting for inventory is very complex

- There are two principal inventory accounting systems:
  - Perpetual inventory systems
  - Periodic inventory systems

McGrawHillIrwin ©The McGraw-Hill Companies, Inc., 2002

Perpetual Inventory Accounting Systems

- A record is made of every purchase and sale

- A continuous record of the quantity and cost of each inventory item is maintained

- Computers and bar codes scanning have aided in the development and use of this system

McGrawHill/Irwin   ©The McGraw-Hill Companies, Inc., 2002

Periodic Inventory Accounting Systems

- A count of the inventory on hand is made periodically

- The cost of the inventory on hand, based on the cost-flow assumption being used, is reported on the balance sheet

- The remainder of the beginning inventory and the purchases are reported on the income statement as cost of goods sold

McGrawHill/Irwin   ©The McGraw-Hill Companies, Inc., 2002

Inventory Terms

- In a merchandising operation, inventory is referred to as "merchandise inventory"

- In a manufacturing operation, there are three categories of inventory:

  - **Raw materials inventory** – raw material used in the manufacturing process
  - **Work in process inventory** – items currently being worked on
  - **Finished goods inventory** – ready to be sold

McGrawHill/Irwin   ©The McGraw-Hill Companies, Inc., 2002

Learning Objective 9

- What are the effects of inventory errors on the balance sheet and income statement?

McGrawHill/Irwin   ©The McGraw-Hill Companies, Inc., 2002

Inventory Errors

- Errors in the amount of ending inventory have a direct dollar-for-dollar effect on cost of goods sold and net income

- If ending inventory is understated, cost of goods sold will be overstated, and net income will be understated

- The effect in the subsequent period will be reversed

McGrawHill/Irwin   ©The McGraw-Hill Companies, Inc., 2002

Balance Sheet Valuation at the Lower of Cost or Market

- This reporting is an application of conservatism

- Market is generally the replacement value

- If market is lower than cost, then a loss is recognized

- The determination may be done on an individual item basis or on the inventory as a whole

McGrawHill/Irwin   ©The McGraw-Hill Companies, Inc., 2002

Learning Objective 10

- What are prepaid expenses, and how are they reported on the balance sheet?

Prepaid Expenses and Other Current Assets

- Prepaid expenses are expenses that have been paid in the current fiscal period but will not be subtracted from revenue until a subsequent fiscal period

- Often referred to as a deferral or deferred charge

- Examples are prepaid insurance, prepaid rent, and office supplies

Deferred Tax Assets

- Arise from differences in the fiscal year in which revenues and expenses are recognized for financial accounting purposes and when they are recognized for income tax determination

- Can have deferred tax assets (expenses recognized for financial purposes before they are recognized for tax purposes) and/or deferred tax liabilities (just the opposite)

CHAPTER 6

ACCOUNTING FOR AND
PRESENTATION OF
PROPERTY, PLANT, AND
EQUIPMENT, AND OTHER
NONCURRENT ASSETS

McGraw-Hill/Irwin   ©The McGraw-Hill Companies, Inc., 2002

Learning Objectives

1. How are the costs of land, buildings, and equipment reported on the balance sheet?
2. How are the terms capitalize and expense used with respect to property, plant, and equipment?
3. What are the alternative methods of calculating depreciation for financial accounting purposes, and what are the relative effects of each on the income statement (depreciation expense) and the balance sheet (accumulated depreciation)?

McGraw-Hill/Irwin   ©The McGraw-Hill Companies, Inc., 2002

Learning Objectives

4. Why is depreciation for income tax purposes an important concern of tax-payers, and how does tax depreciation differ from financial accounting depreciation?
5. What is the accounting treatment of maintenance and repair expenditures?
6. What is the effect on the financial statements of the disposition of noncurrent assets either by abandonment or sale?
7. What is the difference between and operating lease and a capital lease?

McGraw-Hill/Irwin   ©The McGraw-Hill Companies, Inc., 2002

Learning Objectives

8. What are the similarities in the financial statement effects of buying an asset compared to using a capital lease to acquire the rights to an asset?

9. What are the meanings of various intangible assets, how are their values measured, and how are their costs reflected in the income statement?

10. What is the role of present value concepts in financial reporting, and what is their usefulness in decision making?

McGraw-Hill/Irwin   ©The McGraw-Hill Companies, Inc., 2002

Learning Objective 1

- How are the costs of land, buildings, and equipment reported on the balance sheet?

McGraw-Hill/Irwin   ©The McGraw-Hill Companies, Inc., 2002

Land

- Shown on the balance sheet at its original cost

- Cost includes all ordinary and necessary items to get the land ready for its intended use

- Land acquired for investment or potential future use is classified as a noncurrent, nonoperating asset

- Land is not depreciated

- Gains and losses on the sale of land are recognized as the difference between the cost of the land and the amount received

McGraw-Hill/Irwin   ©The McGraw-Hill Companies, Inc., 2002

Learning Objective 2

- How are the terms capitalize and expense used with respect to property, plant, and equipment?

Capitalization

- Expenditures should be capitalized if the item acquired will have an economic benefit beyond the current fiscal year

- Capitalized assets – except land – are depreciated

- Depreciation expense is recognized over the useful life of the asset

- Materiality concept is applied to capitalization

- Accounting judgment plays a role in determination of capitalization

---

Expense

- Expenditures should be expensed if the item acquired will not have an economic benefit beyond the current fiscal year

- Expenditures for preventive maintenance are expensed

- Items are expensed if their costs are not material, even if they have a useful life of several years

Learning Objective 1

- How are the costs of land, buildings, and equipment reported on the balance sheet?

McGraw-Hill/Irwin ©The McGraw-Hill Companies, Inc., 2002

Buildings and Equipment

- Recorded at original cost
- Cost includes all ordinary and necessary costs to get the asset ready to use
- Interest costs associated with the loans used to finance construction are capitalized until the building is put in operation
- Installation costs and shake-down costs are capitalized
- Self-manufactured asset cost includes materials, labor, and overhead costs

McGraw-Hill/Irwin ©The McGraw-Hill Companies, Inc., 2002

Basket Purchase Allocation

- When two or more items are purchased in a single transaction, the cost of each asset must be determined
- The allocation of the purchase price is made based on the relative appraisal values of each asset to the total
- See Exhibit 6-2 in text

McGraw-Hill/Irwin ©The McGraw-Hill Companies, Inc., 2002

Depreciation for Financial Accounting Purposes

- An application of the matching concept since an asset is a prepaid cost

- A portion of the cost should be subtracted from the revenues that are generated through the use of the asset

- Depreciation is the allocation of the cost of an asset to the time periods benefited

McGrawHill/Irwin   ©The McGraw-Hill Companies, Inc., 2002

Recording Depreciation

- The expense "Depreciation Expense" is increased

- The contra asset account "Accumulated Depreciation" is increased

- The journal entry is as follows:

  Depreciation Expense   xx
          Accumulated Depreciation   xx

McGrawHill/Irwin   ©The McGraw-Hill Companies, Inc., 2002

Depreciation Details

- The balance in the **Accumulated Depreciation** account is the cumulative total of all depreciation expense recorded over the life of the asset

- **Net book value** is the cost of the asset less the accumulated depreciation

- Note: cash is not involved in the depreciation entry

McGrawHill/Irwin   ©The McGraw-Hill Companies, Inc., 2002

Learning Objective 3

- What are the alternative methods of calculating depreciation for financial accounting purposes, and what are the relative effects of each on the income statement (depreciation expense) and the balance sheet (accumulated depreciation)?

Depreciation Methods

- **Accelerated depreciation** results in greater depreciation expense and lower net income during the early years of an asset's life

- **Straight-line depreciation** results in even amounts of depreciation being taken over the life of the asset

Depreciation Calculation Methods

- The specific depreciation calculation methods are:
  - Straight-line
  - Units of production
  - Sum-of-the-years'-digits
  - Declining balance

Straight-Line Depreciation

- Annual amount of depreciation is calculated as follows:

Cost – Estimated salvage value
Estimated useful life

- The same amount of depreciation expense is taken each year

McGrawHillIrwin   ©The McGraw-Hill Companies, Inc., 2002

_____

_____

_____

_____

_____

_____

_____

Units-of-Production Depreciation

- The depreciation expense per unit produced is calculated as follows:

Cost – Estimated salvage value
Estimated total units to be made

- The depreciation expense for the period is calculated by multiplying the number of units produced that period times the depreciation expense per unit

McGrawHillIrwin   ©The McGraw-Hill Companies, Inc., 2002

_____

_____

_____

_____

_____

_____

_____

Sum-of-the-Years' Digits Depreciation

- Annual depreciation expense is calculated as follows:

(Cost – Estimated salvage value) x

$$\left[\frac{\text{Remaining life in years}}{\text{Sum-of-the-years' digits}} \right]$$

- Results in greater depreciation expense earlier in the life of the asset

McGrawHillIrwin   ©The McGraw-Hill Companies, Inc., 2002

_____

_____

_____

_____

_____

_____

_____

Declining-Balance Depreciation

- Annual depreciation expense is calculated as follows:

Double the straight-line depreciation rate	X	Asset's net book value at beginning of year

- Greater depreciation expense is taken earlier in the life of the asset

Learning Objective 4

- Why is depreciation for income tax purposes an important concern of taxpayers, and how does tax depreciation differ from financial accounting depreciation?

Depreciation Expense for Income Tax Purposes

- Depreciation is a deductible expense for income tax purposes

- In 1981, ACRS was placed in use

- In 1986, MACRS lengthened the lives of the assets for depreciation purposes and additional categories were added

- Most firms do not use income tax depreciation methods for financial reporting purposes – tax rules are subject to frequent change

Learning Objective 5

- What is the accounting treatment of maintenance and repair expenditures?

McGrawHillIrwin   ©The McGrawHill Companies, Inc., 2002

Maintenance and Repair Expenditures

- Preventative maintenance expenditures and routine repair costs are expenses of the period in which they were incurred

- If a maintenance expenditure will extend the useful life or salvage value of an asset beyond that originally used in the depreciation expense calculation, the expenditure should be capitalized

McGrawHillIrwin   ©The McGrawHill Companies, Inc., 2002

Learning Objective 6

- What is the effect on the financial statements of the disposition of noncurrent assets either by abandonment or sale?

McGrawHillIrwin   ©The McGrawHill Companies, Inc., 2002

Disposal of Depreciable Assets

- When a depreciable asset is sold or scrapped, both the asset and the related accumulated depreciation account must be reduced by the appropriate amounts

- If net book value is greater than amount received, a loss will result

- If net book value is less than the amount received, a gain will result

McGraw-Hill/Irwin   ©The McGraw-Hill Companies, Inc., 2002

Learning Objective 7

- What is the difference between and operating lease and a capital lease?

McGraw-Hill/Irwin   ©The McGraw-Hill Companies, Inc., 2002

Assets Acquired by Capital Lease

- **Operating lease** – just the use of the asset; does not involve any attributes of ownership

- **Capital lease** (financing lease) – lessee (renter) assumes all of the risks and benefits of ownership

McGraw-Hill/Irwin   ©The McGraw-Hill Companies, Inc., 2002

Capital Lease Criteria

- A lease is categorized as a capital lease if **any** of the following apply:
  - The lease transfers ownership of the asset to the lessee
  - The lease permits the lessee to purchase the asset at a nominal price at the end of the lease
  - The lease term is at least 75% of the asset's economic life
  - The present value of the lease payments is at least 90% of the fair value of the asset

McGraw-Hill/Irwin ©The McGraw-Hill Companies, Inc., 2002

Learning Objective 8

- What are the similarities in the financial statement effects of buying an asset compared to using a capital lease to acquire the rights to an asset?

McGraw-Hill/Irwin ©The McGraw-Hill Companies, Inc., 2002

Similarities of Buying and Leasing

- Before the FASB lease standard was issued in 1976, many capital leases were not reported in the financial statements

- Leases not appearing on financial statements is called off-balance-sheet financing

- Now both the asset and the related liability are reported on the balance sheet

McGraw-Hill/Irwin ©The McGraw-Hill Companies, Inc., 2002

Lease Transactions

- A lease payment reduces cash, reduces the lease liability, and increases interest expense:

Interest expense	xx	
Capital lease liability	xx	
Cash		xx

- The leased asset is depreciated:

Depreciation expense	xx	
Accumulated depreciation	xx	

Learning Objective 9

- What are the meanings of various intangible assets, how are their values measured, and how are their costs reflected in the income statement?

Intangible Assets

- Long-lived assets that are represented by a contractual right or result from a purchase transaction

- Is not physically identifiable

- Are amortized – the process of allocating the cost of the intangible asset to expense over time

Examples of Intangible Assets

- **Leasehold improvements –** modification expenses for leased spaces

- **Patents –** licenses granted by the government giving the control of the use or sale of an invention for a period of 17 years

- **Trademarks –** registered with the Federal Trade Commission for an unlimited life

McGrawHillIrwin   ©The McGrawHill Companies, Inc., 2002

_____

_____

_____

_____

_____

_____

_____

More Examples of Intangible Assets

- **Copyrights –** protections granted to writers and artists to prevent unauthorized copying of a work. The protection is granted for the life of the artist or writer plus 50 years

- **Goodwill –** the result of a purchase of one firm by another for a price greater than the fair value of the net assets acquired

McGrawHillIrwin   ©The McGrawHill Companies, Inc., 2002

_____

_____

_____

_____

_____

_____

Natural Resources

- Consist of coal deposits, crude oil reserves, timber, mineral deposits , etc.

- The using up of the natural resource is called depletion

  - The concept of depletion is similar to depreciation, only more complicated
  - Usually computed on a straight-line basis

McGrawHillIrwin   ©The McGrawHill Companies, Inc., 2002

_____

_____

_____

_____

_____

_____

_____

Other Noncurrent Assets

- Long-term investments
- Notes receivable that are due more than one year in the future
- Are reclassified as they become current (receivable within a year)

McGraw-Hill/Irwin   ©The McGraw-Hill Companies, Inc., 2002

Learning Objective 10

- What is the role of present value concepts in financial reporting, and what is their usefulness in decision making?

McGraw-Hill/Irwin   ©The McGraw-Hill Companies, Inc., 2002

Present Value

- An application of compound interest – the process of earning interest on interest
- Involves determining the present amount that is equivalent to an amount to be paid or received in the future
- Recognizes that money does have value over time
- The interest rate is called the discount rate

McGraw-Hill/Irwin   ©The McGraw-Hill Companies, Inc., 2002

Present Value Calculations

- Can use for events that consist of a single payment or a series of payments (called an annuity)

- Formulas and computer programs and calculators can calculate present value

- The appendix demonstrates how to calculate present value using tables containing present value factors

McGrawHill/Irwin   ©The McGraw-Hill Companies, Inc., 2002

CHAPTER 7

ACCOUNTING FOR AND PRESENTATION OF LIABILITIES

McGrawHill/Irwin   ©The McGraw-Hill Companies, Inc., 2002

Learning Objectives

1. What is the financial statement presentation of short-term debt and current maturities of long-term debt?
2. What is the difference between interest calculated on a straight basis and on a discount basis?
3. What are unearned revenues and how are they presented in the balance sheet?

McGrawHill/Irwin   ©The McGraw-Hill Companies, Inc., 2002

Learning Objectives

4. What is the accounting for employer's liability for payroll and payroll taxes?
5. What is the importance of making estimates for certain accrued liabilities and how are these items presented in the balance sheet?
6. What is leverage and how is it provided by long-term debt?
7. What are the different characteristics of a bond?

McGrawHill/Irwin   ©The McGraw-Hill Companies, Inc., 2002

Learning Objectives

8. Why does bond discount or premium arise and how is it accounted for?
9. What are deferred income taxes and why do they arise?
10. What is minority interest, why does it arise, and what does it mean in the balance sheet?

McGrawHillIrwin   ©The McGrawHill Companies, Inc., 2002

Learning Objective 1

- What is the financial statement presentation of short-term debt and current maturities of long-term debt?

McGrawHillIrwin   ©The McGrawHill Companies, Inc., 2002

Current Liabilities

- Amounts due within one year or operating cycle
- A working capital loan is a short-term loan with the expectation that it will be repaid from the collection of accounts receivable generated by the sale of inventory
- A revolving line of credit is a predetermined maximum amount, but flexibility in timing and amount borrowed

McGrawHillIrwin   ©The McGrawHill Companies, Inc., 2002

Notes Payable

- A note is a formal promise to pay a stated amount at a stated date, usually with interest

- Prime rate is the term frequently used to express the interest rate on short-term loans

McGraw-Hill/Irwin   ©The McGraw-Hill Companies, Inc., 2002

Learning Objective 2

- What is the difference between interest calculated on a straight basis and on a discount basis?

McGraw-Hill/Irwin   ©The McGraw-Hill Companies, Inc., 2002

Interest Calculation Methods

- Straight interest is calculated as follows:
  Interest = Principal x Rate x Time (in years)

- A discount is interest that is subtracted from the loan principal and the borrower receives the difference

- The difference received by the borrower is called the proceeds

- The discounted amount is shown in the balance sheet as a contra liability

McGraw-Hill/Irwin   ©The McGraw-Hill Companies, Inc., 2002

Current Maturities of Long-Term Debt

- The portion of long-term borrowing that must be repaid within a year of the balance sheet date is reported as a current liability

- The remainder of the long-term debt is shown in noncurrent liabilities

McGraw-Hill/Irwin   ©The McGraw-Hill Companies, Inc., 2002

Accounts Payable

- Accounts payable are amounts owed to suppliers for goods and services that have been provided to the entity on credit

- May be reported using either the gross or the net method

- The gross method recognizes cash discounts when the invoices are paid within the discount period

- The net method recognizes cash discounts when purchases are made

McGraw-Hill/Irwin   ©The McGraw-Hill Companies, Inc., 2002

Learning Objective 3

- What are unearned revenues and how are they presented in the balance sheet?

McGraw-Hill/Irwin   ©The McGraw-Hill Companies, Inc., 2002

Unearned Revenues or Deferred Credits

- Unearned revenues occur when customers pay for goods or services before the goods or services are delivered:

Cash	xx	
Unearned revenue		xx

- When earned, the liability of unearned revenues is removed and recorded as revenues:

Unearned revenue	xx	
Revenue		xx

McGraw-Hill/Irwin © The McGraw-Hill Companies, Inc., 2002

Learning Objective 4

- What is the accounting for employer's liability for payroll and payroll taxes?

McGraw-Hill/Irwin © The McGraw-Hill Companies, Inc., 2002

Payroll Taxes and Other Withholdings

- **Gross pay** is wages earned by an employee

- **Net pay** is the amount the employee receives after deductions

- **Deductions** include federal income tax, state income tax, FICA withholding, union dues, and many others

McGraw-Hill/Irwin © The McGraw-Hill Companies, Inc., 2002

Liabilities from Withholdings

- Amounts withheld are liabilities to the employer until paid

- Additional liabilities result since employers are subject to federal and state payroll taxes

- These payroll taxes are an expense to the employer

McGraw-Hill/Irwin   ©The McGraw-Hill Companies, Inc., 2002

Other Accrued Liabilities

- There are many other liabilities that are accrued by entities
  - **Accrued property taxes**
  - **Estimated warranty liabilities**
  - **Accrued interest** – if not reported separately

McGraw-Hill/Irwin   ©The McGraw-Hill Companies, Inc., 2002

Learning Objective 5

- What is the importance of making estimates for certain accrued liabilities and how are these items presented in the balance sheet?

McGraw-Hill/Irwin   ©The McGraw-Hill Companies, Inc., 2002

Presentation of Accrued Liabilities

- Estimates of accrued liabilities are presented on the balance sheet as current liabilities since they are due within one year of the balance sheet date

- These estimated items are originally recorded as increases in expenses and increases in liabilities

- Adjustments are made to the liabilities as the actual cost is determined

McGrawHillIrwin   ©The McGraw-Hill Companies, Inc., 2002

Learning Objective 6

- What is leverage and how is it provided by long-term debt?

McGrawHillIrwin   ©The McGraw-Hill Companies, Inc., 2002

Noncurrent Liabilities

- **Capital structure** is the mix of debt and owners' equity used to finance the acquisition of the firm's assets

- Using long-term debt has the advantage of having interest expense being deductible – whereas dividends on stock are not deductible

McGrawHillIrwin   ©The McGraw-Hill Companies, Inc., 2002

Financial Leverage

- Financial leverage is the difference between the rate of return earned on assets (ROI) and the rate of return earned on owners' equity (ROE)

- A firm can borrow money to purchase assets and use those assets to earn a rate of return greater than the interest incurred on the borrowed funds

McGrawHillIrwin   ©The McGraw-Hill Companies, Inc., 2002

Learning Objective 7

- What are the different characteristics of a bond?

McGrawHillIrwin   ©The McGraw-Hill Companies, Inc., 2002

Bonds Payable

- Most long-term debt is issued in the form of bonds

- A bond is a formal debt document usually issued in denominations of $1,000

- Bond prices are expressed as a percentage of the bonds principal amount

McGrawHillIrwin   ©The McGraw-Hill Companies, Inc., 2002

Learning Objective 8

- Why does bond discount or premium arise and how is it accounted for?

Bond Premiums and Bond Discounts

- A bond premium is the excess of a bond's market value over its face amount

- A bond discount is the excess of the face amount over the market value of the bond

- Premiums and discounts usually result from differences between stated interest rates on the bonds and the market rate of interest

Reporting Bonds – At Par

- Issuance of bond:

Cash	XX	
Bonds payable		XX

- Recording interest expense:

Interest expense	XX
Cash	XX

- Retirement of bond:

Bonds payable	XX	
Cash		XX

Reporting Bonds – At Discount

- Issuance of bond:

Cash	XX	
Discount on bonds payable	XX	
Bonds payable		XX

- Recording interest expense:

Interest expense	XX	
Discount on bonds payable		XX
Cash		XX

- Retirement of bond:

Bonds payable	XX	
Cash		XX

McGraw-Hill/Irwin · ©The McGraw-Hill Companies, Inc., 2002

Reporting Bonds – At Premium

- Issuance of bond:

Cash	XX	
Premium on bonds payable		XX
Bonds payable		XX

- Recording interest expense:

Interest expense	XX	
Premium on bonds payable	XX	
Cash		XX

- Retirement of bond:

Bonds payable	XX	
Cash		XX

McGraw-Hill/Irwin · ©The McGraw-Hill Companies, Inc., 2002

Types of Bonds

- **Callable bonds** – the issuer may payoff the bonds before the scheduled maturity date
- **Registered bonds** – the name and address of the bond owner is known to the issuer
- **Coupon bonds** – the owner is not known to the issuer
- **Debenture bonds** – secured only by the general credit of the issuer

McGraw-Hill/Irwin · ©The McGraw-Hill Companies, Inc., 2002

More Types of Bonds

- **Mortgage bonds** – secured by a lien against real estate owned by the issuer

- **Term bonds** – requires a lump-sum payment of the face amount of the bonds at maturity

- **Serial bonds** – repaid in installments

- **Convertible bonds** – may be converted into stock of the issuer corporation at the option of the bondholder

McGraw-Hill/Irwin   ©The McGraw-Hill Companies, Inc., 2002

Learning Objective 9

- What are deferred income taxes and why do they arise?

McGraw-Hill/Irwin   ©The McGraw-Hill Companies, Inc., 2002

Deferred Tax Liabilities

- Deferred tax liabilities are provided for temporary differences between income tax and financial statement recognition of revenues and expenses

- Normally are long-term liabilities

- The most significant temporary difference is related to depreciation expense

- The deferred tax liability is the difference between income tax expense and income tax payable

McGraw-Hill/Irwin   ©The McGraw-Hill Companies, Inc., 2002

Other Noncurrent Liabilities

- Obligations related to **pension plans** are noncurrent liabilities
- Obligations related to **post-retirement benefits**
- Estimated liability under **lawsuits** in progress also may be listed as noncurrent liabilities

Learning Objective 10

- What is minority interest, why does it arise, and what does it mean in the balance sheet?

Minority Interest in Subsidiaries

- A subsidiary is a corporation that is more than 50% owned by the firm for which financial statements have been prepared
- The resulting financial statements are called consolidated financial statements
- Minority interest arises if the subsidiary is not 100% owned by the parent corporation
- The minority is the equity of other shareholders

CHAPTER 8

ACCOUNTING FOR AND PRESENTATION OF OWNERS' EQUITY

McGraw-Hill/Irwin   ©The McGraw-Hill Companies, Inc., 2002

Learning Objectives

- What are the characteristics of common stock, and how is common stock presented in the balance sheet?
- What is preferred stock, what are its advantages and disadvantages to the corporation, and how is it presented on the balance sheet?
- How are cash dividends accounted for, and what are the dates involved in dividend transactions?

McGraw-Hill/Irwin   ©The McGraw-Hill Companies, Inc., 2002

Learning Objectives

- What are stock dividends and stock splits, and why are they used?
- What are the components of "other comprehensive income," and why do these items appear in owners' equity?
- What is treasury stock, why is it acquired, and how do treasury stock transactions affect owners' equity?
- How are owners' equity transactions for the year reported in the financial statements?

McGraw-Hill/Irwin   ©The McGraw-Hill Companies, Inc., 2002

Learning Objective 1

- What are the characteristics of common stock, and how is common stock presented in the balance sheet?

Owners' Equity

- The claim of the entity's owners to the assets shown in the balance sheet

- Also called net assets

- Owner's equity for a individual proprietorship is called proprietor's capital

- Owners' equity of a partnerships is called partners' capital

- Owners' equity for a corporation consists of paid-in capital and retained earnings

---

Paid-In Capital

- Referred to as contributed capital

- Consists of:
  - Common stock
  - Preferred stock
  - Additional paid-in capital

Common Stock

- Also called capital stock

- The ultimate owners of the corporation

- Have claim to all assets after all liabilities and preferred stock claims have been satisfied

- Have the right and obligation to elect members of the corporation's board of directors

McGrawHillIrwin   ©The McGrawHill Companies, Inc., 2002

_____

_____

_____

_____

_____

_____

_____

Value of Common Stock

- Common stock can have par or no-par

- Par value is the nominal value assigned to the stock when the corporation is formed

- Usually a stock cannot be issued for a value less than par

- Stated value stock is essentially the same as par value

McGrawHillIrwin   ©The McGrawHill Companies, Inc., 2002

_____

_____

_____

_____

_____

_____

_____

Recording Common Stock

- Par-value common stock sold above par is recorded as follows:

Cash	xx	
Common stock		xx
Additional paid-in capital		xx

- No-par common stock is recorded as follows:

Cash	xx	
Common stock		xx

McGrawHillIrwin   ©The McGrawHill Companies, Inc., 2002

_____

_____

_____

_____

_____

_____

_____

Common Stock Disclosures

- **Authorized shares** of stock represents the maximum number of shares of stock the corporation is legally approved to issue

- **Issued shares** represents the number of shares of stock that have been transferred from the corporation to shareholders

- **Outstanding shares** of stock represents the shares of stock still in the hands of shareholders

- **Treasury stock** represents the difference between issued and outstanding shares

McGraw-Hill/Irwin   ©The McGraw-Hill Companies, Inc., 2002

Learning Objective 2

- What is preferred stock, what are its advantages and disadvantages to the corporation, and how is it presented on the balance sheet?

McGraw-Hill/Irwin   ©The McGraw-Hill Companies, Inc., 2002

Preferred Stock

- Has several debt-like features and a limited claim on the assets in the event of liquidation

- Most preferred stock receives a quarterly or semiannual dividend

- A dividend is a distribution of earnings of a corporation to its owners

- The amount of the dividend is usually stated as a dollar amount or as a percentage (of par value)

McGraw-Hill/Irwin   ©The McGraw-Hill Companies, Inc., 2002

Preferred Stock Dividends

- A **cumulative dividend** means that a missed dividend must be paid before dividends are paid to common shareholders

- A **participating dividend** means that after common stockholders have received a specified dividend, further dividends are shared by common and preferred shareholders

- A **liquidating dividend** is the preferred stock claim on assets in the event of liquidation

Types of Preferred Stock

- **Callable preferred stock** is redeemable at the option of the corporation

- **Convertible preferred stock** may be exchanged for common stock of the corporation at the option of the shareholder at a stated conversion rate

Additional Paid-In Capital

- The owners' equity category that reflects the excess of the amount received from the sale of preferred or common stock over par value

- Also referred to as capital in excess of par value or capital surplus

Retained Earnings

- The retained earnings account reflects the cumulative earnings of the corporation that have been retained for use in the business rather than paid out as dividends

- Retained earnings are **not** cash

- The main factors affecting retained earnings are net income (or loss) and dividends

---

Learning Objective 3

- How are cash dividends accounted for, and what are the dates involved in dividend transactions?

Cash Dividends

- To pay a dividend, a corporation must have:
  - Sufficient retained earnings
  - Sufficient cash to pay the dividend
  - A dividend declaration by the board of directors

- The key dates related to dividends are:
  - Date of declaration
  - Date of record
  - Date of payment

Dividend Dates

- **Date of declaration** is the date the board of directors declares the dividend

- **Date of record** is the date used to determine who receives the dividend – the stockholders of record as of that date

- **Date of payment** is the date the dividend checks are mailed to the shareholders

- **Ex-dividend date** is three business days before the date of record – the stock trades without the dividend

McGrawHillIrwin   ©The McGraw-Hill Companies, Inc., 2002

Learning Objective 4

- What are stock dividends and stock splits, and why are they used?

McGrawHillIrwin   ©The McGraw-Hill Companies, Inc., 2002

Stock Dividends

- The issuance of additional stock to existing shareholders in proportion to the number of shares currently owned

- Used to maintain loyalty of stockholders when the firm does not have enough cash for a cash dividend

- Affects only owners' equity of the firm:

Retained earnings	**XX**
Common stock	**XX**
Additional paid-in capital	**XX**

McGrawHillIrwin   ©The McGraw-Hill Companies, Inc., 2002

Stock Split

- Will lower the market price of a firm's stock

- Involves issuing additional share of stock to existing shareholders

- No accounting entry is required

- The par value and the number of shares issued changes

McGrawHill/Irwin · ©The McGraw-Hill Companies, Inc., 2002

Learning Objective 6

- What is treasury stock, why is it acquired, and how do treasury stock transactions affect owners' equity?

McGrawHill/Irwin · ©The McGraw-Hill Companies, Inc., 2002

Treasury Stock

- Shares of a corporation's own stock that have been purchased from shareholders

- Is reflected on the balance sheet as a contra owners' equity account

- Treasure stock is **not** an asset

- Recorded as follows:

Treasury stock	xx	
Cash		xx

McGrawHill/Irwin · ©The McGraw-Hill Companies, Inc., 2002

Sales of Treasury Stock

- When sold above purchase price, treasury stock transactions are recorded as follows:

Cash	**XX**	
Treasury stock		**XX**
Additional paid-in capital		**XX**

- Cash dividends are not paid on treasury stock since the firm would be paying itself a dividend

- Stock dividends and stock splits do affect treasury stock

McGraw-Hill/Irwin ©The McGraw-Hill Companies, Inc., 2002

Learning Objective 5

- What are the components of "other comprehensive income," and why do these items appear in owners' equity?

McGraw-Hill/Irwin ©The McGraw-Hill Companies, Inc., 2002

Other Comprehensive Income

- All items of income (or loss) ultimately affect owners' equity

- Comprehensive income consists of:
  - Net income (from income statement)
  - Cumulative foreign currency translation adjustment
  - Unrealized gains and losses on available-for-sale securities (after taxes)
  - Additional minimum pension liability adjustments (after taxes)

McGraw-Hill/Irwin ©The McGraw-Hill Companies, Inc., 2002

Cumulative Foreign Currency Translation Adjustment

- Financial statements of a foreign subsidiary are expressed in the currency of the country in which it operates

- The financial statements must be converted into U.S. dollars

- Because of fluctuations in exchange rates, a difference occurs between the translated assets and liabilities and the translated owners' equity

McGrawHillIrwin   ©The McGrawHill Companies, Inc., 2002

Cumulative Foreign Currency Translation Adjustment

- The difference may result in a gain or loss

- The adjustment will fluctuate over time and will not be realized until the subsidiary is sold

McGrawHillIrwin   ©The McGrawHill Companies, Inc., 2002

Learning Objective 7

- How are owners' equity transactions for the year reported in the financial statements?

McGrawHillIrwin   ©The McGrawHill Companies, Inc., 2002

Reporting Changes in Owners' Equity Accounts

- May be reported in the balance sheet, a separate statement of changes in owners' equity, or in the footnotes or financial review accompanying the financial statements

- Reports all changes in owners' equity for the year

Owners' Equity for Other Types of Entities

- Proprietorships and partnership do not issue stock

- No distinction is made between paid-in capital and retained earnings

- Distributions made to owners are usually recorded in a drawing account – similar to a dividend account

Owners' Equity for Other Types of Entities

- Not-for-profit and governmental entities do not have owners who have a direct financial interest in the entity

- Owners' equity is referred to as fund balance

- A statement of changes in fund balances takes the place of a statement of owners' equity

CHAPTER 9

THE INCOME STATEMENT AND THE STATEMENT OF CASH FLOWS

McGrawHill/Irwin ©The McGraw-Hill Companies, Inc., 2002

Learning Objectives

1. What is revenue, and what are the two criteria that permit revenue recognition?
2. How is cost of goods sold determined under both perpetual and periodic inventory accounting systems?
3. What is the significance of gross profit, and how is gross profit calculated and used?
4. What are the principal categories and components of "other operating expenses," and how are these items reported on the income statement?

McGrawHill/Irwin ©The McGraw-Hill Companies, Inc., 2002

Learning Objectives

5. What is included in "income from operations," and why is this income statement subtotal significant to managers and financial analysts?
6. What are the components of the earnings per share calculation, and what are the reasons for some of the refinements made in that calculation?
7. What are the alternative income statement presentation models?

McGrawHill/Irwin ©The McGraw-Hill Companies, Inc., 2002

Learning Objectives

8. What are the unusual items that may appear on the income statement?
9. What are the purpose and general format of the statement of cash flows?
10. What is the difference between the direct and the indirect methods of presenting cash flows from operating activities?
11. Why is the statement of cash flows significant to financial analysts and investors who rely on the financial statements?

Learning Objective 1

- What is revenue, and what are the two criteria that permit revenue recognition?

Income Statement

- Answers important questions such as:
  - What are the financial results of operations of the entity for the fiscal year?
  - Are sales increasing relative to cost of goods sold and other operating expenses?
- Reports what has happened over a period of time

Revenues

- Inflows or other enhancements of assets from rendering goods or services that constitute the entity's ongoing, major operations
- To be recognized, revenue must be:
  - **Realized or realizable**
  - **Earned**

Realization and Earned

- **Realization** – the product or service has been exchanged for cash or claims to cash
- **Earned** – the entity has completed the activities it must perform to be entitled to the revenue benefits
- Both criteria are usually satisfied when product being sold is delivered to the customer

Sales

- **Sales** – describes the revenues of firms that sell purchased or manufactured products
- **Sales returns and allowances** – a refund or reduced price for defective merchandise
- **Net sales** – gross sales less sales returns and allowances
- Other terms for revenues include Rental Revenue, Fees, and Other Revenues

Shipping Terms

- **FOB destination** – the seller owns the product until accepted by the buyer at the buyer's designated location. Title to the merchandise passes when the merchandise is received by the buyer. Seller incurs shipping costs

- **FOB shipping point** – buyer accepts ownership of the product at the seller's shipping location. Buyer incurs shipping costs.

Gains

- Increases in net assets resulting from incidental transactions or nonoperating activities

- Not included with revenues at the beginning of the income statement

- Reported as "other income"

Expenses

- Outflows or other using up of assets or incurrence of liabilities from delivering goods or services that constitute the entity's ongoing, major operations

- Based on the matching principle

- Some recognized in the period in which they are incurred (administrative expenses)

- Others are an allocation of cost (depreciation)

Losses

- Decreases in an entity's net assets resulting from incidental transactions or nonoperating activities

- Not included with expenses on the income statement

- Reported after "income from operations"

McGrawHillIrwin   ©The McGrawHill Companies, Inc., 2002

Learning Objective 2

- How is cost of goods sold determined under both perpetual and periodic inventory accounting systems?

McGrawHillIrwin   ©The McGrawHill Companies, Inc., 2002

Cost of Goods Sold

- Most significant expense for many manufacturing and merchandising firms

- Inventory shrinkage usually included
- Is a function of the inventory cost flow assumption

- Computed as (under periodic system):

- **Cost of beginning inventory + Net purchases – Cost of ending inventory**

McGrawHillIrwin   ©The McGrawHill Companies, Inc., 2002

Net Purchases

- Purchases are the inventory bought for resale in a merchandising firm

- Freight charges are added

- Purchase discounts are deducted

- Purchase returns and allowances – refunds or credits for defective merchandise – are deducted

McGraw-Hill/Irwin   ©The McGraw-Hill Companies, Inc., 2002

Expanded Cost of Goods Sold

Cost of beginning inventory		xx
+ Purchases	xx	
+ Freight charges	xx	
- Purchase discounts	xx	
- Purchase returns and allowances	xx	
Net purchases		xx
= Cost of goods available for sale		xx
- Cost of ending inventory		xx
= Cost of goods sold		xx

McGraw-Hill/Irwin   ©The McGraw-Hill Companies, Inc., 2002

Learning Objective 3

- What is the significance of gross profit, and how is gross profit calculated and used?

McGraw-Hill/Irwin   ©The McGraw-Hill Companies, Inc., 2002

Gross Profit or Gross Margin

- The difference between sales revenue and cost of goods sold

- May be expressed as a dollar amount or as a percentage of sales (**gross profit ratio**)

- A measure of the amount of each sales dollar that is available to cover operating expenses and profit

- Can be used to estimate cost of good sold and ending inventory when physical inventory has not been taken

McGrawHillIrwin   ©The McGrawHill Companies, Inc., 2002

Gross Profit Ratio

- Gross profit divided by sales

- Can be used to set selling prices

- Differs by class of merchandise sold

- Sales mix is the proportion of sales of each class of merchandise

- Overall gross profit ratio depends on the sales mix

McGrawHillIrwin   ©The McGrawHill Companies, Inc., 2002

Learning Objective 4

- What are the principal categories and components of "other operating expenses," and how are these items reported on the income statement?

McGrawHillIrwin   ©The McGrawHill Companies, Inc., 2002

Other Operating Expenses

- Consists of:
  - Selling expenses
  - General and administrative expenses
  - Research and development expenses
- Footnotes to the financial statements often offer details about these expenses

McGrawHill/Irwin ©The McGraw-Hill Companies, Inc., 2002

Learning Objective 5

- What is included in "income from operations," and why is this income statement subtotal significant to managers and financial analysts?

McGrawHill/Irwin ©The McGraw-Hill Companies, Inc., 2002

Income From Operations

- The difference between gross profit and operating expenses
- Most appropriate measure of management's ability to utilize the firm's operating assets
- Excludes interest expense, interest income, gains and losses, income taxes, and other nonoperating transactions

McGrawHill/Irwin ©The McGraw-Hill Companies, Inc., 2002

Other Income and Expenses

- Includes interest expense, interest income, gains, and losses
- Items that are not significant are reported in "other income" and "other expenses"
- Nonoperating gains and losses include sale or disposal of assets, losses from inventory obsolescence, and litigation gains and losses

---

Income Before Income Taxes

- Listed on the income statement after other income and expenses
- Listed before income tax expense
- Usually a footnote to the financial statements discloses detail of the income tax calculation

---

Net Income

- Net income is often referred to as "the bottom line"
- All revenues and gains less all expenses and losses
- Since net income impacts dividends, stockholders and potential investors are very interested in net income

Learning Objective 6

- What are the components of the earnings per share calculation, and what are the reasons for some of the refinements made in that calculation?

Earnings Per Share

- Used to facilitate interpretation of net income
- **Basic earnings per share** is net income divided by the weighted average number of shares of common stock outstanding
- **Diluted earnings per share** also is shown if a firm has convertible securities

Calculation of Earnings Per Share

- Basic earnings per share =

$$\frac{\text{Net income} - \text{preferred stock dividends}}{\text{Weighted average number of common shares outstanding}}$$

- The weighting of the shares outstanding is done based on the number of months each block of shares has been outstanding

Other Earnings Per Share Amounts

- If any securities (bonds or preferred stock) are convertible to common stock, diluted earnings per share is reported

- In this calculation, it is assumed that the securities have been converted and the dividends or interest have not been paid

- Earnings per share also is shown for any unusual items on the income statement

McGraw-Hill/Irwin   ©The McGraw-Hill Companies, Inc., 2002

_____

_____

_____

_____

_____

_____

Learning Objective 7

- What are the alternative income statement presentation models?

McGraw-Hill/Irwin   ©The McGraw-Hill Companies, Inc., 2002

_____

_____

_____

_____

_____

_____

Income Statement Presentation Alternatives

- **Single step format** uses no breakdowns as to gross profit, operating income, etc.

- All items are listed in order with no subtotals in the single step format

- **Multiple step format** uses subtotals and categories of income and expenses

McGraw-Hill/Irwin   ©The McGraw-Hill Companies, Inc., 2002

_____

_____

_____

_____

_____

_____

Learning Objective 8

- What are the unusual items that may appear on the income statement?

McGraw-Hill/Irwin   ©The McGraw-Hill Companies, Inc., 2002

Unusual Items Sometimes Seen on an Income Statement

- Income statements are used by investors to predict probable results of future operations, but they only want to consider recurring items

- Nonrecurring items are reported separately, net of the income tax effect of the event

- These events include: discontinued operations, extraordinary items, minority interest in subsidiaries, and cumulative effect of change in accounting principle

McGraw-Hill/Irwin   ©The McGraw-Hill Companies, Inc., 2002

Discontinued Operations

- Disclose the impact of a the disposal of a segment or major portion of a business

- Helps investors see the impact on the firm's operations without the disposed business segment

- Shown net of taxes

- Report earnings per share effect of disposal

McGraw-Hill/Irwin   ©The McGraw-Hill Companies, Inc., 2002

Extraordinary Items

- Must be unusual in nature and infrequent in occurrence to qualify as an extraordinary item (or if prescribed by the FASB)

- The event is not likely to recur

- Examples include: gains and losses from early repayment of long-term debt, litigation settlements, and pension plan terminations

- Shown net of tax

- Report earnings per share for extraordinary items

McGraw-Hill/Irwin   ©The McGraw-Hill Companies, Inc., 2002

Minority Interest in Earnings of Subsidiaries

- The financial statements of a subsidiary are combined with those of the parent

- Only the parent's equity in the subsidiary's earnings is reported

- The minority interest earnings are deducted from income after taxes

- Reported separately only if significant

McGraw-Hill/Irwin   ©The McGraw-Hill Companies, Inc., 2002

Cumulative Effect of a Change in Accounting Principle

- A change from one generally accepted accounting principle to another is permitted only if the change is promulgated by a standard-setting body or if the change can be justified

- Report the cumulative effect of the change net of tax

McGraw-Hill/Irwin   ©The McGraw-Hill Companies, Inc., 2002

Learning Objective 9

- What are the purpose and general format of the statement of cash flows?

Statement of Cash Flows

- Relatively new financial statement
- Primary purpose is to provide relevant information about the cash receipts and cash payments of an entity during a period
- Key word is "cash"

Learning Objective 10

- What is the difference between the direct and the indirect methods of presenting cash flows from operating activities?

Cash Flows from Operating Activities

- Two methods of presenting the operating activities section:
  - The **direct method** involves listing each major class of cash receipts and cash disbursements
  - The **indirect method** explains cash flow by explaining the change in each of the non-cash operating accounts in the balance sheet

McGraw-Hill/Irwin ©The McGraw-Hill Companies, Inc., 2002

Direct Method

- Lists cash activities such as:
  - Cash received from customers
  - Cash paid to merchandise or raw materials suppliers
  - Cash paid to employees for wages
  - Cash paid for interest
  - Cash paid for income taxes

McGraw-Hill/Irwin ©The McGraw-Hill Companies, Inc., 2002

Indirect Method

- Begins with net income and adds back depreciation expense
- Adjusts for changes in non-cash operating accounts in the balance sheet such as accounts receivable, inventory, and accounts payable
- Also need to include deferred income taxes, gains and losses on assets, and amortization on bonds payable

McGraw-Hill/Irwin ©The McGraw-Hill Companies, Inc., 2002

Cash Flows from Investing and Financing Activities

- Investing activities relate to the purchase and sale of noncurrent assets such as land and buildings and debt and equity securities

- Financing activities relate to changes in noncurrent liabilities and owners' equity accounts such as issuing bonds or stock and paying dividends

McGraw-HillIrwin   ©The McGrawHill Companies, Inc., 2002

Learning Objective 11

- Why is the statement of cash flows significant to financial analysts and investors who rely on the financial statements?

McGraw-HillIrwin   ©The McGrawHill Companies, Inc., 2002

Interpreting the Statement of Cash Flows

- Did the firm's cash balance increase or decrease during the period?

- A firm should have a positive cash flow from operating activities

- Cash from operating activities should be greater than cash used for investing activities

- Can often determine a firm's growth strategy from the statement of cash flows

McGraw-HillIrwin   ©The McGrawHill Companies, Inc., 2002

CHAPTER 10

EXPLANATORY NOTES AND OTHER FINANCIAL INFORMATION

McGraw-Hill/Irwin   ©The McGraw-Hill Companies, Inc., 2002

Learning Objectives

1. Are the explanatory notes an integral part of the financial statements? Do the notes provide detailed disclosure needed by users wishing to gain a full understanding of the financial statements?

2. What are the kinds of significant accounting policies that are explained in the notes?

McGraw-Hill/Irwin   ©The McGraw-Hill Companies, Inc., 2002

Learning Objectives

3. What are the nature and content of disclosures relating to accounting changes, business combinations, contingencies and commitments, events subsequent to the balance sheet date, impact of inflation, and segment information?

4. What is the role of the Securities and Exchange Commission, and what are some of its reporting requirements?

McGraw-Hill/Irwin   ©The McGraw-Hill Companies, Inc., 2002

Learning Objectives

5. Why is a statement of management's responsibility included with the notes?
6. What is the significance of management' discussion and analysis of the firm's financial condition and results of operations?
7. What is included in the five-year (or longer) summary of financial information?
8. What are the meaning and content of the independent auditor's report?

McGraw-Hill/Irwin   ©The McGraw-Hill Companies, Inc. 2002

Learning Objective 1

• Are the explanatory notes an integral part of the financial statements? Do the notes provide detailed disclosure needed by users wishing to gain a full understanding of the financial statements?

McGraw-Hill/Irwin   ©The McGraw-Hill Companies, Inc. 2002

General Organization

• The explanatory notes refer to specific items in the financial statements

• The financial statement sequence is usually as follows:
  – Income statement
  – Balance Sheet
  – Statement of cash flows

• The placement of the statement of changes in owners' equity depends on the complexity of the statement

McGraw-Hill/Irwin   ©The McGraw-Hill Companies, Inc. 2002

Explanatory Notes

- **Full disclosure** requires that firms report all information necessary for a reasonably astute user not to be misled

- Explanatory notes generally require more pages than the statements themselves

McGraw-Hill/Irwin ©The McGraw-Hill Companies, Inc., 2002

Learning Objective 2

- What are the kinds of significant accounting policies that are explained in the notes?

McGraw-Hill/Irwin ©The McGraw-Hill Companies, Inc., 2002

Significant Accounting Policies

- Management may choose from a number of choices among generally accepted accounting practices

- Each firm must disclose the policies chosen

- Disclosure enables users to make intelligent comparisons among firms

McGraw-Hill/Irwin ©The McGraw-Hill Companies, Inc., 2002

Types of Significant Accounting Policies

- **Depreciation method** – method used and useful lives are disclosed

- **Inventory valuation method** – methods for each category of inventory are disclosed. If LIFO used, the difference between it and what inventory would have been under FIFO is disclosed

- **Basis of consolidation** – discloses which subsidiaries are consolidated, if any

McGraw-Hill/Irwin   ©The McGraw-Hill Companies, Inc., 2002

More Types of Significant Accounting Policies

- **Income taxes** – a reconciliation of the statutory rate and the effective tax rate is provided. An explanation of deferred taxes also is included

- **Employee benefits** – the cost of employee benefit is disclosed, along with actuarial assumptions

- **Amortization of intangible assets** – method of amortization is disclosed

McGraw-Hill/Irwin   ©The McGraw-Hill Companies, Inc., 2002

More Types of Significant Accounting Policies

- **Earnings per share of common stock** – an explanation of the calculation is provided

- **Stock option** and **stock purchase plans** – officers and key employees are given the right to purchase stock at some time in the future. Details of such plans are provided

McGraw-Hill/Irwin   ©The McGraw-Hill Companies, Inc., 2002

Details of Other Financial Statement Amounts

- May include the amount of research and development expenses

- May include what items are included in the "other income" category

- Details of long-term debt may be provided

- Details of other costs and expenses

McGraw-Hill/Irwin   ©The McGraw-Hill Companies, Inc., 2002

Learning Objective 3

- What are the nature and content of disclosures relating to accounting changes, business combinations, contingencies and commitments, events subsequent to the balance sheet date, impact of inflation, and segment information?

McGraw-Hill/Irwin   ©The McGraw-Hill Companies, Inc., 2002

Other Disclosures

- **Accounting change** – a change in accounting principle that has a material effect on the comparability of the current period with prior periods. Example: changing from FIFO to LIFO

- **Business combinations** – the effect on the financial statements from mergers, acquisitions, or dispositions will be reported

McGraw-Hill/Irwin   ©The McGraw-Hill Companies, Inc., 2002

More Disclosures

- **Contingencies and commitments** – firms involved in lawsuits must disclose the facts of the lawsuit. Must also disclose if a guarantor of the indebtedness of another entity

- **Events subsequent to the balance sheet date** – a significant event that will materially impact the financial statement s must be disclosed

©The McGraw-Hill Companies, Inc., 2002

McGraw-Hill/Irwin

More Disclosures

- **Impact of inflation** – a firm must report the effect of inflation on the financial statements

- **Segment information** – must disclose line of business and geographic segment operating profit, capital expenditures, depreciation and amortization, identifiable assets, and sales to unaffiliated customers

©The McGraw-Hill Companies, Inc., 2002

McGraw-Hill/Irwin

Learning Objective 4

- What is the role of the Securities and Exchange Commission, and what are some of its reporting requirements?

©The McGraw-Hill Companies, Inc., 2002

McGraw-Hill/Irwin

Reporting to the Securities and Exchange Commission

- The SEC was created to administer securities laws
- Securities that are offered for sale to more than a few investors must be registered with the SEC
- A prospectus is provided to investors prior to their purchase of securities
- Firms must file annual reports, 10-Ks, with the SEC

McGraw-Hill/Irwin ©The McGraw-Hill Companies, Inc., 2002

Learning Objective 5

- Why is a statement of management's responsibility included with the notes?

McGraw-Hill/Irwin ©The McGraw-Hill Companies, Inc., 2002

Management's Statement of Responsibility

- Explains that the responsibility for the financial statements lies with the management of the firm
- Usually refers to the firm' internal control, the internal audit function, the audit committee of the board of directors, and other ethical conduct matters

McGraw-Hill/Irwin ©The McGraw-Hill Companies, Inc., 2002

Learning Objective 6

- What is the significance of management' discussion and analysis of the firm's financial condition and results of operations?

Management's Discussion and Analysis

- A discussion by management of the firm's activities during the year, its financial condition, and the results of operations

- Required by the SEC in annual reports to them, but now included in most firm's annual reports to stockholders

Learning Objective 7

- What is included in the five-year (or longer) summary of financial information?

Five-Year (or Longer) Summary of Financial Data

- Includes key income statement data

- Includes significant ratios such as earnings as a percent of sales

- Includes earnings and dividends per share

- May include stock prices

McGraw-Hill/Irwin ©The McGraw-Hill Companies, Inc., 2002

Learning Objective 8

- What are the meaning and content of the independent auditor's report?

McGraw-Hill/Irwin ©The McGraw-Hill Companies, Inc., 2002

Independent Auditors' Report

- Brief (usually three paragraphs) report
- Usually addressed to board of directors and stockholders
- Identifies the statements that were audited
- Describes the nature and extent of the auditors' work
- Contains an opinion about fair presentation
- Contains the name of the audit firm and a signature

McGraw-Hill/Irwin ©The McGraw-Hill Companies, Inc., 2002

Financial Statement Compilations

- A report that states that the financial statements have not been audited

- Does not provide any assurance as to the fairness of the financial statements

- Less costly than an audit

McGraw-Hill/Irwin   ©The McGraw-Hill Companies, Inc., 2002

CHAPTER 11

FINANCIAL STATEMENT ANALYSIS

McGraw-Hill/Irwin   ©The McGraw-Hill Companies, Inc., 2002

_____

_____

_____

_____

_____

_____

_____

Learning Objectives

1. How can liquidity measures be influenced by the inventory cost-flow assumption used?
2. How do suppliers and creditors use a customer's payment practices to judge liquidity?
3. What are the influences of alternative inventory cost-flow assumptions and depreciation methods on turnover ratios?

McGraw-Hill/Irwin   ©The McGraw-Hill Companies, Inc., 2002

_____

_____

_____

_____

_____

_____

Learning Objectives

4. How are the number of days' sales in accounts receivable and inventory used to evaluate the effectiveness of the management of receivables and inventory?
5. What is the significance of the price/earnings ratio in the evaluation of the market price of a company's stock?

McGraw-Hill/Irwin   ©The McGraw-Hill Companies, Inc., 2002

_____

_____

_____

_____

_____

_____

Learning Objectives

6. How are dividend yield and the dividend payout ratio used by investors to evaluate a company's common stock?
7. What is financial leverage, and why is it significant to management, creditors, and owners?
8. What is book value per share of common stock, how is it calculated, and why is it not a very meaningful amount for most companies?

Learning Objectives

9. How can common size financial statements be used to evaluate a firm's financial position and results of operations over a number of years?
10. How can operating statistics using physical, or non-financial data, be used to help management evaluate the results of the firm's activities?

Learning Objective 1

- How can liquidity measures be influenced by the inventory cost-flow assumption used?

Financial Statement Analysis Ratios

- Used to facilitate the interpretation of an entity' financial position and results of operations

- Can be classified into four groups:
  - Liquidity
  - Activity
  - Profitability
  - Debt, or financial leverage

Liquidity Measures

- The balance sheet carrying values of inventory will depend on the cost-flow assumption used
- Cannot compare firms using different inventory cost-flow assumptions
- Firms often report the LIFO reserve – the difference between LIFO an FIFO inventory values

Liquidity Ratios

- Working capital =

  Current assets – Current liabilities

- Current ratio = $\dfrac{\text{Current assets}}{\text{Current liabilities}}$

- Acid-test ratio =

  $\dfrac{\text{Cash + Accounts receivable}}{\text{Current liabilities}}$

Learning Objective 2

- How do suppliers and creditors use a customer's payment practices to judge liquidity?

Customer's Payment Practices

- Suppliers and creditors want to know if a firm is paying its bills promptly

- This information may be obtained from other suppliers, credit bureaus, and Dun & Bradstreet reports

- Credit bureaus and credit rating agencies provide a graded rating for firms

Learning Objective 3

- What are the influences of alternative inventory cost-flow assumptions and depreciation methods on turnover ratios?

Activity Measures

- Focus primarily on the relationship between assets and sales

- In computing activity measures, average assets is used

- Average asset amounts include inventory and fixed assets

- The values of inventory (based on cost-flow assumptions) and fixed assets (based on book cost less accumulated depreciation) depend on the cost-flow assumptions and depreciation methods used

McGraw-Hill/Irwin   ©The McGraw-Hill Companies, Inc., 2002

_____

_____

_____

_____

_____

_____

Activity Ratios

- Total asset turnover = $\dfrac{\text{Sales}}{\text{Average total assets}}$

- Inventory turnover = $\dfrac{\text{Cost of goods sold}}{\text{Average inventories}}$

- Number of days' sales in accounts receivable = $\dfrac{\text{Accounts receivable}}{\text{Average days' sales}}$

McGraw-Hill/Irwin   ©The McGraw-Hill Companies, Inc., 2002

_____

_____

_____

_____

_____

_____

More Activity Ratios

- Average days' sales = $\dfrac{\text{Annual sales}}{365}$

- Number of days' sales in inventory =

  $\dfrac{\text{Inventory}}{\text{Average days' cost of goods sold}}$

- Average days' cost of goods sold =

  $\dfrac{\text{Average cost of goods sold}}{365}$

McGraw-Hill/Irwin   ©The McGraw-Hill Companies, Inc., 2002

_____

_____

_____

_____

_____

_____

Learning Objective 4

- How are the number of days' sales in accounts receivable and inventory used to evaluate the effectiveness of the management of receivables and inventory?

Number of Days' Sales in Accounts Receivable

- Assesses the efficiency of managing accounts receivable
- The sooner accounts receivable are collected, the sooner cash is available for use in the business
- Generally, the higher the turnover and lower the number in days' sales, the better
- An increase in the age of accounts receivable is a warning that profitability and liquidity may be weakening

---

Number of Days' Sales in Inventory

- Assesses the efficiency of managing inventory
- The lower that inventories can be maintained relative to sales, the less inventory that needs to be financed with debt and the greater the return on investment
- Trend in the efficiency of managing inventory is the important factor

Profitability Measures

- Operating income is frequently used in ROI calculations because it is a more direct measure of management's activities

- Average ROI based on net income for most American firms is between 7% and 10%

- Again, trends are important

Profitability Ratios

- ROI =

$$\frac{\text{Return (Net income)}}{\text{Investment (Average total assets)}}$$

- DuPont model =

Margin	x	Turnover
$\dfrac{\text{Net income}}{\text{Sales}}$	x	$\dfrac{\text{Sales}}{\text{Average total assets}}$

More Profitability Ratios

- ROE = $\dfrac{\text{Net income}}{\text{Average total owners' equity}}$

- Dividend yield = $\dfrac{\text{Annual dividend per share}}{\text{Market price per share of stock}}$

- Dividend payout ratio = $\dfrac{\text{Annual dividend per share}}{\text{Earnings per share}}$

Learning Objective 5

- What is the significance of the price/earnings ratio in the evaluation of the market price of a company's stock?

McGrawHillIrwin ©The McGrawHill Companies, Inc., 2002

Price/Earning Ratio

- P/E ratio =

  Market price of a share of common stock
  Earnings per share of common stock

- Used extensively to evaluate the market price of a firm's common stock relative to that of other firms and the market as a whole
- Also called **earnings multiple**

McGrawHillIrwin ©The McGrawHill Companies, Inc., 2002

Importance of P/E Ratio

- Investors can earn a return on stock two ways:
  - Through dividends
  - Through increases in the market value of the stock
- Market price reflects expectations of future dividends – which depend on earnings
- Typically, manufacturing firms' P/E ratio ranges from 12 to 18

McGrawHillIrwin ©The McGrawHill Companies, Inc., 2002

Learning Objective 6

- How are dividend yield and the dividend payout ratio used by investors to evaluate a company's common stock?

Dividend Yield

- Dividend yield =

Annual dividend per share
Market price per share of stock

- Should be compared to the yield available on other investments

- On common stock, historically this has ranged from 3% to 6%

- On preferred stock, the range is 5% to 8%

Dividend Payout Ratio

- Dividend payout ratio =

Annual dividend per share
Earnings per share

- Reflects the dividend policy of the firm

- Most firms pay a relatively constant portion of earnings and avoid fluctuations

- Generally, ranges from 30% to 50% for manufacturing and merchandising firms

Preferred Dividend Coverage Ratio

- Preferred dividend coverage ratio =

  Net income
  Preferred dividend requirement

- Indicates the margin of safety of the preferred stock dividend

Learning Objective 7

- What is financial leverage, and why is it significant to management, creditors, and owners?

Financial Leverage Measures

- Refers to the use of debt to finance the assets of the entity

- Adds risk to the operation of the firm

- Also magnifies the return to owners relative to the return on assets

- Firms want to borrow at a rate less than the rate of return on financed assets

- Interest is a deductible expense; dividends are not deductible

Debt Ratio

- Indicates the extent to which a firm is using financial leverage

- Debt ratio =

  Total liabilities
  Total liabilities and owners' equity

- Indicates the percentage of financing that is done with debt

---

Debt/Equity Ratio

- Another indicator of the extent to which a firm is using financial leverage

- Debt/Equity ratio =   **Total liabilities**
  Total owners' equity

- Indicates the percentage of financing that is done with debt

- Since deferred taxes and current liabilities are not interest bearing, these items are often excluded from the computation

---

Times Interest Earned Ratio

- A measure that shows the relationship of earnings before interest and taxes to interest expense

- The greater the ratio, the more confident the debt holders are about the firm continuing to earn enough to cover interest payments

- Times interest earned =

  Earnings before interest and taxes
  Interest expense

Learning Objective 8

- What is book value per share of common stock, how is it calculated, and why is it not a very meaningful amount for most companies?

Book Value per Share of Common Stock

- Easily misunderstood

- Cannot be compared to market value due to book value reflects the application of generally accepted accounting principles and the specific accounting policies that the firm has selected

- Book value per share of common stock =

  $$\frac{\text{Common shareholders' equity}}{\text{Number of shares of common stock outstanding}}$$

Learning Objective 9

- How can common size financial statements be used to evaluate a firm's financial position and results of operations over a number of years?

Common Size Financial Statements

- Used when evaluating the operating results of a firm over a number of years

- Each asset, liability, and owners' equity account is expressed as a percentage of total assets

- On the income statement, sales is set at 100%, and each item is expressed as a percentage of sales

McGrawHillIrwin   ©The McGrawHill Companies, Inc., 2002

Use of Common Size Financial Statements

- Using percentages makes spotting trends easier

- Can compare firms of different sizes

- In horizontal analysis, several years' financial data are stated in terms of a base year

- Each item in the base year is 100%; the items in subsequent years are a percentage of the item in the base year

McGrawHillIrwin   ©The McGrawHill Companies, Inc., 2002

Learning Objective 10

- How can operating statistics using physical, or non-financial data, be used to help management evaluate the results of the firm's activities?

McGrawHillIrwin   ©The McGrawHill Companies, Inc., 2002

Other Operating Statistics

- Physical measures also are useful

- Sales in units removes hidden price changes

- Total employees may be more useful than payroll costs

- Usually analysts combine financial and physical measures to show trends and to make comparisons

CHAPTER 12

MANAGERIAL ACCOUNTING AND COST-VOLUME-PROFIT RELATIONSHIPS

McGraw-Hill/Irwin   ©The McGraw-Hill Companies, Inc., 2002

Learning Objectives

1. What is the managerial planning and control cycle?
2. What are the major differences between financial accounting and managerial accounting?
3. What is the difference between variable and fixed cost behavior patterns, and what simplifying assumptions are made in this classification method?

McGraw-Hill/Irwin   ©The McGraw-Hill Companies, Inc., 2002

Learning Objectives

4. Why are fixed costs expressed on a per unit of activity basis misleading, and why may this result in faulty decisions?
5. What kinds of costs are likely to have a variable cost behavior pattern, and what kinds of costs are likely to have a fixed costs behavior pattern?
6. How can the high-low method be used to determine the cost formula for a cost that has a mixed behavior pattern?

McGraw-Hill/Irwin   ©The McGraw-Hill Companies, Inc., 2002

Learning Objectives

7. What is the difference between the traditional income statement format and the contribution statement format?

8. What is the importance of using the contribution margin format to analyze the impact of cost and sales volume changes on operating income?

9. How is the contribution margin ratio calculated, and how can it be used in CVP analysis?

McGrawHill/Irwin   ©The McGraw-Hill Companies. Inc., 2002

Learning Objectives

10. How can changes in sales mix affect the projections using CVP analysis?

11. What are the meaning and significance of the break-even point, and how is the break-even point calculated?

12. What is the concept of operating leverage?

McGrawHill/Irwin   ©The McGraw-Hill Companies. Inc., 2002

Learning Objective 1

• What is the managerial planning and control cycle?

McGrawHill/Irwin   ©The McGraw-Hill Companies. Inc., 2002

Managerial Accounting Contrasted to Financial Accounting

- **Managerial accounting** supports the internal planning decision made by management

- **Financial accounting** has more of a score-keeping, historical orientation

- Planning is a key part of the management process

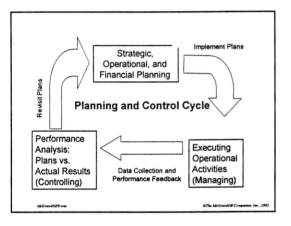

Planning and Control

- The management process consists of planning, organizing, and controlling an entity's activities

- Control provides feedback in which actual results are compared to planned results, and if a variance exists, the plan or actions or both are changed

Learning Objective 2

- What are the major differences between financial accounting and managerial accounting?

McGrawHillIrwin   ©The McGrawHill Companies, Inc., 2002

Managerial Accounting

- Emphasis is on the future
- Concerned with units within the organization
- Reports issued frequently and promptly
- Relevance more important than reliability
- No reporting standards
- Intended to management's use

McGrawHillIrwin   ©The McGrawHill Companies, Inc., 2002

Financial Accounting

- Intended for external investors and creditors
- Deals with the past – historical
- Reports are prepared for the company as a whole
- Reports are issued monthly – a week or more after the end of the month
- High accuracy is desired
- Generally Accepted Accounting Standards are used for reports

McGrawHillIrwin   ©The McGrawHill Companies, Inc., 2002

The Management Accountant

- Works extensively with people in other functions of the organization

- Helps develop production standards

- Helps production people interpret production reports

- Helps marketing and sales predict future sales

- Aids in the information system development

McGrawHillIrwin   ©The McGrawHill Companies, Inc., 2002

Learning Objective 3

- What is the difference between variable and fixed cost behavior patterns, and what simplifying assumptions are made in this classification method?

McGrawHillIrwin   ©The McGrawHill Companies, Inc., 2002

Cost Classifications

- Different costs for different purposes:

  - Relationship between total cost and volume of activity

  - Relationship to product or activity

  - For cost accounting purposes

  - Time frame perspective

  - Other analytical purposes

- These classifications are not mutually exclusive

McGrawHillIrwin   ©The McGrawHill Companies, Inc., 2002

Relationship of Total Cost to Volume of Activity

- The relationship of total cost to volume of activity describes the cost behavior pattern

- A variable cost changes in TOTAL as the volume of activity changes

- A fixed cost does NOT change in TOTAL as the volume of activity changes

- Variable cost example is raw materials

- Fixed cost example is depreciation

McGraw-Hill/Irwin   ©The McGraw-Hill Companies, Inc., 2002

Graphical Representation

Variable costs   **Fixed costs**

Total activity (units)   Total activity (units)

McGraw-Hill/Irwin   ©The McGraw-Hill Companies, Inc., 2002

Semivariable Costs

- Some costs have components of both fixed and variable costs

- A cost formula for such a cost is:
  Total cost = **Fixed cost + Variable cost**
  or
  Total cost = **Fixed cost + (Variable rate per unit X Activity)**

McGraw-Hill/Irwin   ©The McGraw-Hill Companies, Inc., 2002

Learning Objective 4

- Why are fixed costs expressed on a per unit of activity basis misleading, and why may this result in faulty decisions?

McGrawHillIrwin   ©The McGrawHill Companies, Inc., 2002

Fixed Cost Unitization

- Do NOT unitize fixed expenses because they do not behave on a per unit basis

- Dividing fixed expenses by activity level will give varying results depending on the activity level

McGrawHillIrwin   ©The McGrawHill Companies, Inc., 2002

Learning Objective 5

- What kinds of costs are likely to have a variable cost behavior pattern, and what kinds of costs are likely to have a fixed cost behavior pattern?

McGrawHillIrwin   ©The McGrawHill Companies, Inc., 2002

Cost Behavior Pattern

- Two assumptions made in determining cost behavior patterns:
  - The behavior pattern is true only within a relevant range
  - The behavior pattern is assumed to be linear in the relevant range
- The relevant range is the level of activity over which a particular pattern exists

Learning Objective 6

- How can the high-low method be used to determine the cost formula for a cost that has a mixed behavior pattern?

The High-Low Method

- A cost behavior pattern can be analyzed using a technique that employs a scattergram to identify high and low cost-volume data
- A scattergram is a graph with total units produced as the horizontal axis and cost as the vertical axis
- Points are plotted on the graph for various production levels and costs

Steps in Using the High-Low Method

1. Identify·the high and low cost-volume points
2. Compute the variable rate by using the following formula:

Variable rate =
$$\frac{\text{High cost} - \text{Low cost}}{\text{High activity} - \text{Low activity}}$$

McGrawHillIrwin   ©The McGrawHill Companies, Inc., 2002

Steps in Using the High-Low Method

3. Compute the fixed rate by using the following formula and inserting the variable rate computed above and either the high activity level or the low activity level

   Total cost = **Fixed cost + Variable cost**
   Total cost = **Fixed cost + (Activity level x Variable rate)**

McGrawHillIrwin   ©The McGrawHill Companies, Inc., 2002

Learning Objective 7

- What is the difference between the traditional income statement format and the contribution statement format?

McGrawHillIrwin   ©The McGrawHill Companies, Inc., 2002

Modified Income Statement Format

- Referred to as the contribution margin format

- Classifies costs according to their behavior

- Revenues and operating income are the same as under the traditional format of revenues minus cost of goods sold, etc.

Contribution Margin Format

- Revenues   XX
  - Variable expenses   XX
  - = Contribution margin   XX
  - Fixed expenses   XX
  - = Operating income   XX

Learning Objective 8

- What is the importance of using the contribution margin format to analyze the impact of cost and sales volume changes on operating income?

Contribution Margin

- Contribution margin is the amount that is available to cover fixed expenses and operating income

- The traditional approach does not consider cost behavior patterns

- The contribution margin approach avoids the errors that may result from viewing fixed costs on a per unit approach

McGrawHillIrwin   ©The McGrawHill Companies, Inc., 2002

Learning Objective 9

- How is the contribution margin ratio calculated, and how can it be used in CVP analysis?

McGrawHillIrwin   ©The McGrawHill Companies, Inc., 2002

Contribution Margin Ratio

- Contribution margin ratio is the ratio of contribution margin to revenues

- Using either total dollars or dollars per unit, divide the contribution margin by the revenue

- The result is a percentage

McGrawHillIrwin   ©The McGrawHill Companies, Inc., 2002

Contribution Margin Model

	Per unit X Volume = Total %
Revenue	$XX
Variable expenses	XX
Contribution margin	$XX x XX = $XX X%
Fixed expenses	XX
Operating income	$XX

McGrawHillIrwin   ©The McGrawHill Companies, Inc., 2002

Using the Contribution Margin Model

- Steps in using the model are as follows:

  - Express revenue, variable expense, and contribution on a per unit basis

  - Multiply the contribution per unit by the volume to get the total contribution margin

  - Subtract fixed expenses from the total contribution margin to get operating income (Fixed expenses are NOT unitized!)

McGrawHillIrwin   ©The McGrawHill Companies, Inc., 2002

Contribution Margin in Action

- Four relationships to notice as you study:

  - Revenue - Variable expenses = **Contribution margin**

  - Contribution margin / Revenue = **Contribution margin ratio**

  - Total contribution margin depends on the volume of activity

  - Contribution margin must cover fixed expenses before an operating income is earned

McGrawHillIrwin   ©The McGrawHill Companies, Inc., 2002

Learning Objective 10

- How can changes in sales mix affect the projections using CVP analysis?

McGrawHillIrwin   ©The McGraw-Hill Companies, Inc., 2002

Multiple Products and Sales Mix Considerations

- When using the contribution margin model with more than one product, the sales mix must be considered

- **Sales mix** is the relative proportion of total sales accounted for by different products

- Different products usually have different contribution margins

McGrawHillIrwin   ©The McGraw-Hill Companies, Inc., 2002

Learning Objective 11

- What are the meaning and significance of the break-even point, and how is the break-even point calculated?

McGrawHillIrwin   ©The McGraw-Hill Companies, Inc., 2002

Break-Even Point Analysis

- **Break-even point** is usually expressed as the amount of revenue that must be realized in order to have neither a profit nor a loss

- Expresses minimum target revenue

- Use the contribution margin model to determine the break-even point by setting operating income to zero

McGraw-Hill/Irwin   ©The McGraw-Hill Companies, Inc., 2002

Break-Even Point Formulas

- Total revenues at break-even =

    Fixed expenses
    Contribution margin ratio

- Volume in units at bread-even =

    Fixed expenses
    Contribution margin per unit

- Volume in units at break-even =

    Total revenues required
    Revenue per unit

McGraw-Hill/Irwin   ©The McGraw-Hill Companies, Inc., 2002

Target Operating Income

- The revenues and units necessary may be determined as follows:

- Total revenues for desired level of operating income =

- **Fixed expenses + Desired operating income**
    Contribution margin ratio

- Volume in units for desired level of operating income =

- **Fixed expenses + Desired operating income**
    Contribution margin per unit

McGraw-Hill/Irwin   ©The McGraw-Hill Companies, Inc., 2002

Break-Even Graph

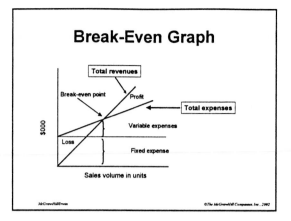

Total revenues

Break-even point

Profit

Total expenses

Variable expenses

Loss

Fixed expense

$000

Sales volume in units

Learning Objective 12

- What is the concept of operating leverage?

Operating Leverage

- Operating income will change proportionately more than changes in revenues because fixed expenses do not change with changes in volume

- This magnification effect on operating income due to a change in revenues is called operating leverage

Operating Leverage Effects

- The higher a firm's contribution margin ratio, the greater its operating leverage

- High operating leverage increases the risk that a small percentage decline in revenues will cause a large percentage decline in operating income

McGrawHillIrwin   ©The McGrawHill Companies, Inc., 2002

CHAPTER 13

COST ACCOUNTING AND REPORTING SYSTEMS

McGrawHillIrwin   ©The McGrawHill Companies, Inc., 2002

Learning Objectives

1. What is the role of cost accounting as it relates to financial and managerial accounting?
2. How does cost management play a strategic role in the organization's value chain?
3. What is the difference between direct and indirect costs, and how do they relate to a product or activity?

McGrawHillIrwin   ©The McGrawHill Companies, Inc., 2002

Learning Objectives

4. What is the difference between product costs and period costs, and what are the three components of product cost?
5. What is the general operation of a product costing system, and how do costs flow through the inventory accounts to cost of goods sold?
6. How are predetermined overhead application rates developed and used?

McGrawHillIrwin   ©The McGrawHill Companies, Inc., 2002

Learning Objectives

7. What is the presentation and interpretation of a statement of cost of goods manufactured?
8. What is the difference between absorption and direct (or variable) costing?
9. What are activity based costing and activity based management?

Learning Objective 1

- What is the role of cost accounting as it relates to financial and managerial accounting?

Cost Accounting

- **Cost accounting** is a subset of managerial accounting
- Deals primarily with the accumulation and determination of product, process, or service costs
- The primary purpose is income measurement and inventory valuation in accordance with generally accepted accounting principles for external financial reporting

Uses of Costing Systems

- Need accurate costing information for:
  - Pricing decisions
  - Evaluating productivity and efficiency
  - Developing operating budgets
  - Determining which product parts will be manufactured internally
  - Analyzing production technology
  - Appraising performance

McGraw-Hill/Irwin   ©The McGraw-Hill Companies, Inc., 2002

Learning Objective 2

- How does cost management play a strategic role in the organization's value chain?

McGraw-Hill/Irwin   ©The McGraw-Hill Companies, Inc., 2002

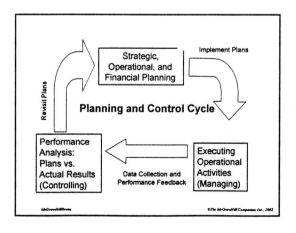

McGraw-Hill/Irwin   ©The McGraw-Hill Companies, Inc., 2002

Cost Management

- **Cost management** is the process of using cost information from the accounting system to manage the activities of the organization

- Accurate and timely information is critical to the success of the decision-making process

- An organization's **value chain** is the sequence of functions and related activities that adds value for the customer

Value Chain Functions

- Research and Development – cost of generating new ideas

- Design – can we make a product at a reasonable cost?

- Production – cost of making the product

- Marketing – cost of promoting the product

- Distribution – cost of delivery

- Customer service – cost of after-sales support

Cost Accumulation and Assignment

- Costs are incurred in carrying out each activity in the value chain

- A **cost object** is a reference point (job, machine, product line, etc.) where a need to understand costs exists

- **Cost accumulation** is the process of collecting and recording transaction data

- **Cost assignment** is the process of attributing an appropriate amount of cost in the cost pool to each cost object

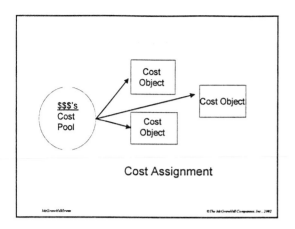

Cost Assignment

Learning Objective 3

- What is the difference between direct and indirect costs, and how do they relate to a product or activity?

Cost Relationship to Product or Activity

- Direct cost and indirect cost classifications depends on the context

- A **direct cost** is a cost that would NOT be incurred if the product or activity were discontinued

- An **indirect cost** is one that would continue to be incurred even if the product or activity were discontinued

Learning Objective 4

- What is the difference between product costs and period costs, and what are the three components of product cost?

McGraw-Hill/Irwin
©The McGraw-Hill Companies, Inc., 2002

Costs for Cost Accounting Purposes

- **Product costs** are used in manufacturing and merchandising firms to determine inventory values
  - Raw materials
  - Direct labor
  - Manufacturing overhead
- **Period costs** as those costs not included in inventory as product costs
- Period costs are reported on the income statement as they are incurred

McGraw-Hill/Irwin
©The McGraw-Hill Companies, Inc., 2002

Product Costs

- **Raw materials** – the ingredients of a product
- **Direct labor** – the effort provided by workers who are directly involved with the manufacture of the product
- **Manufacturing overhead** – includes all manufacturing costs except raw materials and direct labor

McGraw-Hill/Irwin
©The McGraw-Hill Companies, Inc., 2002

Learning Objective 5

- What is the general operation of a product costing system, and how do costs flow through the inventory accounts to cost of goods sold?

McGrawHillIrwin   ©The McGrawHill Companies, Inc., 2002

Cost Accounting Systems

- Every manufacturing firm uses a cost accounting system to accumulate the cost of products made

- The system involves three inventory accounts:
  - Raw material inventory
  - Work in process inventory
  - Finished goods inventory

McGrawHillIrwin   ©The McGrawHill Companies, Inc., 2002

Inventory Accounts

- **Raw materials** – cost of parts used in the manufacturing process

- **Work in process** – used to accumulate all manufacturing costs (raw materials, direct labor, manufacturing overhead) while the product is in processing

- **Finished goods** – cost of goods completed

McGrawHillIrwin   ©The McGrawHill Companies, Inc., 2002

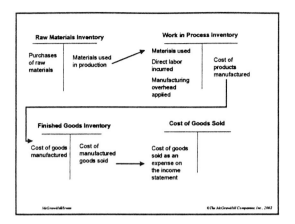

Learning Objective 6

- How are predetermined overhead application rates developed and used?

Overhead Application

- **Manufacturing overhead** is all costs of a product except raw materials and direct labor

- Assigning overhead costs presents a challenge

- Most systems apply overhead by using a single, or few, surrogate measures of overhead behavior

- The assumption is that since products are being made, overhead costs are being incurred

Overhead Application Bases

- An estimate of total overhead is made a the beginning of the year
- A base is selected to apply overhead
  - Direct labor hours
  - Direct labor dollars
  - Machine hours
  - The estimated overhead cost is divided by the total estimated base for the year – thus producing an overhead rate

McGraw-Hill/Irwin   ©The McGraw-Hill Companies, Inc., 2002

_____

_____

_____

_____

_____

_____

_____

Overhead Application Rates

- The overhead application rate may be stated in dollars - $6.00 per machine hour used
- The overhead application rate may be stated in percentages – 130% of direct labor dollars
- These overhead rates are assigned to the costs of the products produced

McGraw-Hill/Irwin   ©The McGraw-Hill Companies, Inc., 2002

_____

_____

_____

_____

_____

_____

Differences Between Actual and Applied Overhead

- The overhead rate is multiplied by the actual base used during the year
- Any difference between the total applied overhead and the actual cost of overhead is transferred to cost of goods sold if immaterial
- If the difference is material, the difference is divided between cost of goods sold and ending inventory

McGraw-Hill/Irwin   ©The McGraw-Hill Companies, Inc., 2002

_____

_____

_____

_____

_____

_____

Learning Objective 7

- What is the presentation and interpretation of a statement of cost of goods manufactured?

McGraw-Hill/Irwin   ©The McGraw-Hill Companies, Inc., 2002

Statement of Cost of Goods Manufactured

- Manufacturing costs are summarized and reported in the statement of cost of goods manufactured

- **Total manufacturing costs** include:
  - Raw materials used
  - Direct labor cost incurred
  - Manufacturing overhead applied

McGraw-Hill/Irwin   ©The McGraw-Hill Companies, Inc., 2002

Statement of Cost of Goods Manufactured – Continued

- Total manufacturing costs incurred are added to beginning work in process inventory

- Then ending work in process inventory is subtracted to arrive at cost of goods manufactured

McGraw-Hill/Irwin   ©The McGraw-Hill Companies, Inc., 2002

Firm XYZ
Statement of Cost of Goods Manufactured
For the Month of XX

Raw Materials:		
Inventory, Beginning	$XX	
Purchases for the month	XX	
Raw materials available for use	$XX	
Less: Inventory, Ending	XX	
Cost of raw materials used		$XX
Direct labor costs incurred for the month		XX
Manufacturing overhead applied for the month		XX
Total manufacturing cost for the month		$XX
Add: Work in process, beginning		XX
Less: Work in process, ending		XX
Cost of goods manufactured for the month		$XX

McGraw-Hill/Irwin ©The McGraw-Hill Companies, Inc., 2002

Cost of Goods Sold

- Cost of goods manufactured is added to beginning finished goods inventory to arrive at cost of goods available for sale

- Ending finished goods inventory is subtracted from cost of goods available for sale to arrive at cost of goods sold

McGraw-Hill/Irwin ©The McGraw-Hill Companies, Inc., 2002

Firm XYZ
Statement of Cost of Goods Sold
For the Month of XX

Beginning inventory	$XX
Cost of goods manufactured	XX
Cost of goods available for sale	$XX
Less: Ending inventory	XX
Cost of goods sold	$XX

McGraw-Hill/Irwin ©The McGraw-Hill Companies, Inc., 2002

Firm XYZ
Income Statement
For the Month of XX

Sales	$XX
Cost of goods sold	XX
Gross profit	$XX
Selling, general, and admin. expenses	XX
Income from operations	$XX
Interest expense	XX
Income before taxes	$XX
Income tax expense	XX
Net income	$XX

Cost Accounting Systems

- **Job order costing systems** are used when discrete products are manufactured

- Costs are accumulated for each job in a job order system

- **Process costing systems** are used when producing homogeneous products

- Costs are accumulated by department in a process costing system

Equivalent Units of Production

- In a process costing system, costs are accumulated by department

- The costs of the department are divided by the equivalent units processed by that department to find a cost per unit

- The **equivalent units of production** is the number of units that would have been produced if all production efforts had resulted in complete products

Learning Objective 8

- What is the difference between absorption and direct (or variable) costing?

McGrawHill/Irwin   ©The McGraw-Hill Companies, Inc., 2002

_____

_____

_____

_____

_____

_____

_____

Absorption Costing and Direct Costing

- In **absorption costing** systems, all manufacturing costs incurred are absorbed into the product cost

- **Direct costing** (or variable costing) assigns only variable costs to products

- In direct costing, fixed manufacturing overhead is treated as an operating expense

- Absorption costing must be used for financial reporting and tax purposes

McGrawHill/Irwin   ©The McGraw-Hill Companies, Inc., 2002

_____

_____

_____

_____

_____

_____

Learning Objective 9

- What are activity based costing and activity based management?

McGrawHill/Irwin   ©The McGraw-Hill Companies, Inc., 2002

_____

_____

_____

_____

_____

_____

_____

Activity-Based Costing

- Overhead costs have become increasing significant due to technological innovations

- As a result, overhead application rates have been applied using activity-based costing

- In **activity-based costing**, an activity must be identified that causes the incurrence of a cost

McGrawHillIrwin   ©The McGrawHill Companies, Inc., 2002

Cost Drivers

- Examples of cost drivers include:
  - Machine setup
  - Quality inspection
  - Production order preparation
  - Materials handling activities

- Activity-based costing is a complex process

- Activity-based costing had led to more accurate costing

McGrawHillIrwin   ©The McGrawHill Companies, Inc., 2002

Activity-Based Management

- **Activity-based management** is the use of activity-based costing information to support the decision making process

- Can be relevant to customer satisfaction, operational productivity and efficiency, product or process design, product mix

- Activity-based management has led to better decisions

McGrawHillIrwin   ©The McGrawHill Companies, Inc., 2002

CHAPTER 14

COST ANALYSIS FOR PLANNING

McGrawHillIrwin ©The McGraw-Hill Companies, Inc., 2002

Learning Objectives

1. What is the cost terminology that relates to the budgeting process?
2. Why are budgets useful, and how does management philosophy influence the budget process?
3. How are alternative budget time frames used?
4. What is the significance of the sales forecast (or revenue budget) to the overall operating budget?

McGrawHillIrwin ©The McGraw-Hill Companies, Inc., 2002

Learning Objectives

5. How is the purchases/production budget developed?
6. What is the importance of cost behavior patterns in developing the operating expense budget?
7. Why are a budgeted income statement and balance sheet prepared?
8. How is the cash budget developed?

McGrawHillIrwin ©The McGraw-Hill Companies, Inc., 2002

Learning Objectives

9. Why and how are standards useful in the planning and control process?
10. How is the standard cost of a product developed?
11. How are standard costs used in the cost accounting system?

Learning Objective 1

- What is the cost terminology that relates to the budgeting process?

Planning and Budgeting

- **Planning** is the initial part of the planning and control cycle

- A **budget** is a plan in financial terms

- The results of an organization's activities will be reported in terms of income, cash flow, and financial position – the financial statements

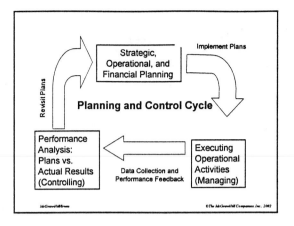

Planning and Control Cycle

Strategic, Operational, and Financial Planning

Implement Plans

Revisit Plans

Performance Analysis: Plans vs. Actual Results (Controlling)

Data Collection and Performance Feedback

Executing Operational Activities (Managing)

Usefulness of Budgets

- The preparation of a budget forces management to plan

- The budget provides a benchmark against which to compare actual performance

- The budgeting process requires communication and coordination among functional areas of a firm

---

Standard Costs

- A **standard cost** is a budget for each component – materials, labor, and overhead – of a product

- Standard costs are used in the planning and control processes of manufacturing and other types of companies

Cost Classifications

- Classifying costs based on the relationship of total cost to volume of activity results in categories of variable, fixed, and mixed costs

- Classifying costs according to a time-frame perspective results in committed and discretionary costs

  - A **committed cost** is incurred to execute a long- range policy decision

  - A **discretionary cost** is one that can be adjusted in the short term at management's discretion

---

Learning Objective 2

- Why are budgets useful, and how does management philosophy influence the budget process?

The Budgeting Process in General

- In a highly structured organization, the budget is seen as carved in stone

- Management philosophy is reflected in whether the budget is prepared using a top-down, dictated, approach or a participative, managers involved, approach

- Most budgets are based on current budgets with revisions
  - the incremental approach

Learning Objective 3

- How are alternative budget time frames used?

The Budget Time Frame

- Budgets can be prepared for a single period or for several periods

- A single-period budget is prepared in the months preceding the beginning of the year and is used the entire year

- A multi-period or rolling budget involves planning for segments of a year on a repetitive basis

- The advantage of a continuous budget is that it will be more accurate, but it takes more effort

---

The Budgeting Process

- First, develop and communicate assumptions about the economy, the industry, and the organization's strategy

- The **operating budget** is made up of a number of detailed budgets:
  - **Sales/revenue budget**
  - **Purchases/production budget**
  - **Operating expense budget**
  - **Income statement budget**
  - **Cash budget**
  - **Balance sheet budget**

Learning Objective 4

- What is the significance of the sales forecast (or revenue budget) to the overall operating budget?

Sales Forecast

- The sales forecast is the key to developing a reasonable budget

- The most challenging component since there is so little control over the variables that influence sales

- Need to consider the past experience of managers, production capacity, pricing policy, and advertising effectiveness

- The other budgeted items are a function of the sales budget

Learning Objective 5

- How is the purchases/production budget developed?

Purchases/Production Budget

- By using the cost of goods sold model with units, the quantity of merchandise to be manufactured or purchased can be determined – after the sales budget

- The firm's inventory policy determines the amounts to be used in the computation

- The inventory policy should take into consideration such factors as lead time and forecast errors

- The ending inventory for one period is the beginning inventory for the next period

McGraw-Hill/Irwin ©The McGraw-Hill Companies, Inc., 2002

Budget Calculations as a Guide

- If a production budget calls for vastly different quantities to be manufactured each period, the production may be planned at a constant level

- If materials can be purchased in certain quantities, the purchase quantities nearest to the calculated value will be used

- Budget calculations provide a guide to action – not absolute amounts

McGraw-Hill/Irwin ©The McGraw-Hill Companies, Inc., 2002

Cost of Goods Sold Budget

- Once the sales budget and the purchases/production budgets have been prepared, the cost of goods sold budget can be prepared

- **Cost of goods sold** consists of:
  - Raw materials budget
  - Direct labor budget
  - Overhead budget

McGraw-Hill/Irwin ©The McGraw-Hill Companies, Inc., 2002

Learning Objective 6

- What is the importance of cost behavior patterns in developing the operating expense budget?

Operating Expense Budget

- Some operating expenses are variable expenses:
  - Sales commissions
- Some operating expenses are fixed:
  - Depreciation
- Therefore, operating expenses are budgeted according to their cost behavior patterns
- Budget slack occurs when managers larger budgets than necessary

---

Learning Objective 7

- Why are a budgeted income statement and balance sheet prepared?

Budgeted Income Statement

- Use the sales forecast, the cost of goods sold budget, and the operating expense budget to prepare budgeted income statement

- An important step in determining profitability and overall satisfactory results

McGraw-Hill/Irwin   ©The McGraw-Hill Companies, Inc., 2002

Budgeted Balance Sheet

- A budgeted balance sheet is prepared after the impact of all the other budgets has been determined

- Depreciation, amortization, inventory, cash, liabilities, and owners' equity are all affected by the other budgets

McGraw-Hill/Irwin   ©The McGraw-Hill Companies, Inc., 2002

Learning Objective 8

- How is the cash budget developed?

McGraw-Hill/Irwin   ©The McGraw-Hill Companies, Inc., 2002

Cash Budget

- Like a budgeted cash flow statement – but with a short time frame

- Must anticipate short-term borrowing needs

- Must know when excess cash can be invested for interest revenue

- Must make assumptions about collection of accounts receivable and sales through a cash receipts budget

- Must make assumptions about cash payments

Learning Objective 9

- Why and how are standards useful in the planning and control process?

Standard Costs

- Used in:
  - Planning and control process of management
  - Value inventory for financial reporting

- Has two inputs:
  - Quantity of input
  - Cost per unit of input

- Is a unit budget

Using Standard Costs

- **Standard costs** are used to compare to actual costs

- Differences are called **variances**

- The variances may be due to either differences in input quantity or differences in cost per input unit

- Appropriately developed, standard costs can be used in the cost accounting system

McGraw-Hill/Irwin ©The McGraw-Hill Companies, Inc., 2002

Learning Objective 10

- How is the standard cost of a product developed?

McGraw-Hill/Irwin ©The McGraw-Hill Companies, Inc., 2002

Developing Standards

- **Ideal standards** – assumes operating conditions will be ideal; maximum efficiency at all times; usually will have unfavorable variances

- **Attainable standards** – recognizes there will be some operating inefficiencies; will have both favorable and unfavorable variances

- **Past experience standards** – includes all inefficiencies from past operations; does not contain a challenge

McGraw-Hill/Irwin ©The McGraw-Hill Companies, Inc., 2002

Learning Objective 11

- How are standard costs used in the cost accounting system?

Costing Products with Standard Costs

- Must aggregate the individual standard costs for each of the inputs:
  - Raw materials
  - Direct labor
  - Overhead

- Purchasing agent provides information about materials costs

- Human resources will provide information about labor costs

Overhead Standard Costs

- Overhead costs are classified as fixed or variable

- Variable overhead will be expressed in terms that reflect the causes of overhead expenditures

- Fixed overhead will be expressed as a total cost per accounting period and allocated to individual products

Other Uses of Standards

- Can be used for planning and control of period costs

- Can be used with quantitative goals of the organization

- The development of goals can be expressed as standards

- Do not have to be expressed in dollars

McGraw-Hill/Irwin   ©The McGraw-Hill Companies, Inc., 2002

Budgeting for Other Analytical Purposes

- Service firms can use budgeting techniques for financial and nonfinancial resources such as time budgets

- Can also be used in manufacturing firms in areas not related to production such as customer service

McGraw-Hill/Irwin   ©The McGraw-Hill Companies, Inc., 2002

CHAPTER 15

COST ANALYSIS FOR CONTROL

McGraw-Hill/Irwin ©The McGraw-Hill Companies, Inc., 2002

Learning Objectives

1. Why are all costs controllable by someone at some time, but in the short run some costs may be classified as noncontrollable?
2. How does performance reporting facilitate the management-by-exception process?
3. How can the operating results of segments of an organization be reported most meaningfully?

McGraw-Hill/Irwin ©The McGraw-Hill Companies, Inc., 2002

Learning Objectives

4. What is a flexible budget, and how is it used?
5. How and why are the two components of a standard cost variance calculated?
6. What are the specific names assigned to variances for different product inputs?

McGraw-Hill/Irwin ©The McGraw-Hill Companies, Inc., 2002

Learning Objectives

7. How do the control and analysis of fixed overhead variances and variable cost variances differ?
8. What are the alternative methods of accounting for variances?

McGraw-Hill/Irwin   ©The McGraw-Hill Companies, Inc., 2002

Learning Objective 1

- Why are all costs controllable by someone at some time, but in the short run some costs may be classified as noncontrollable?

McGraw-Hill/Irwin   ©The McGraw-Hill Companies, Inc., 2002

Performance Reporting

- Involves the comparison of actual results with planned results
- The objective is highlighting those activities where planned and actual results differ
- Appropriate actions may be taken to address the causes of the favorable or unfavorable variances

McGraw-Hill/Irwin   ©The McGraw-Hill Companies, Inc., 2002

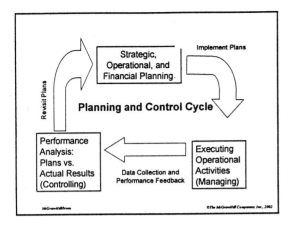

_____

_____

_____

_____

_____

_____

_____

Relationship of Total Costs +/- to Volume of Activity

- Any differences between achieved and planned performances should be evaluated

- As the level of activity changes from the planned activity, total variable costs should change

- The total amount of fixed costs should not change with changes in levels of activity

_____

_____

_____

_____

_____

_____

_____

Cost Classification According to a Time-Frame Perspective

- A **noncontrollable cost** is one which the manager can do nothing to influence the amount of the cost

- Noncontrollable costs occur in the short run

- In the long run every cost is **controllable** by someone in the organization

_____

_____

_____

_____

_____

_____

_____

Learning Objective 2

- How does performance reporting facilitate the management-by-exception process?

McGrawHillIrwin   ©The McGraw-Hill Companies, Inc., 2002

Characteristics of the Performance Report

- A **performance report** compares actual results to budgeted amounts

- It is an integral part of the control process

- The general format is as follows:

	Budget	Actual		
Activity	**Amount**	**Amount**	**Variance**	**Explanation**

McGrawHillIrwin   ©The McGraw-Hill Companies, Inc., 2002

+/-   Variances

- Variances are usually described as either favorable or unfavorable

- A **favorable variance** occurs when results exceed planned activities in a positive manner – revenues are larger than expected

- An **unfavorable variance** occurs when results exceed planned activities in a negative manner – expenses are larger than expected

McGrawHillIrwin   ©The McGraw-Hill Companies, Inc., 2002

Responsibility Reporting

- The explanation column in the performance report is to communicate to upper-level management the causes of variances

- In responsibility reporting, higher levels of management receive less details regarding lower levels in the chain of command

- Managers want to eliminate unfavorable variances and retain favorable variances

McGraw-Hill/Irwin   ©The McGraw-Hill Companies, Inc., 2002

Management by Exception

- Managers concentrate their efforts only on those activities that are not performing according to the plan

- To aid in this effort, variances are often expressed in percentages

- Only those variances that exceed a predetermined percentage are investigated

McGraw-Hill/Irwin   ©The McGraw-Hill Companies, Inc., 2002

Frequency of Performance Reports

- Performance reports should be issued soon after the period in which the activity takes place

- If later, actions are forgotten or confused

- A question regarding performance reports is whether noncontrollable expenses should be reported

- May want managers to be aware of all costs, or may want managers to deal only with controllable costs

McGraw-Hill/Irwin   ©The McGraw-Hill Companies, Inc., 2002

Learning Objective 3

- How can the operating results of segments of an organization be reported most meaningfully?

McGraw-Hill/Irwin ©The McGraw-Hill Companies, Inc., 2002

Reporting for Segments of an Organization

- A **segment** is a division, product line, or other organizational unit

- Using the contribution margin format, sales, variable expenses, contribution margin, fixed expenses, and operating income are calculated for each segment

- Fixed expenses should be divided into direct fixed expenses and common fixed expenses

McGraw-Hill/Irwin ©The McGraw-Hill Companies, Inc., 2002

Segment Fixed Expenses

- Direct fixed expenses would be eliminated if the segment were eliminated

- Common fixed expenses are an allocated portion of the organization's fixed expenses

- Common fixed expenses would not be eliminated if the segment were eliminated

McGraw-Hill/Irwin ©The McGraw-Hill Companies, Inc., 2002

Types of Segments

- A **responsibility center** is an element of the organization over which a manager has responsibility and authority
  - **Cost center** – does not generate revenue for the organization
  - **Profit center** – generates revenue for the organization
  - **Investment center** – generates revenue and controls assets of the organization

---

Evaluating Segments

- Cost centers are evaluated by comparing actual costs incurred to budgeted costs

- Profit centers are evaluated by comparing actual segment margin to budgeted segment margin

- Investment centers are evaluated by comparing actual and budgeted return on investment based on segment margin and assets controlled by the segment

---

Learning Objective 4

- What is a flexible budget, and how is it used?

Flexible Budget

- A **flexible budget** is one that reflects budgeted amounts for actual activity

- Flexible budgeting does not affect the predetermined overhead application rate

- Therefore, fixed overhead will be overapplied or underapplied

Learning Objective 5

- How and why are the two components of a standard cost variance calculated?

Analysis of Variable Cost Variances

- The total variance for a cost component is called the **budget variance**

- The budget variance is caused by two factors:

  – The difference between the standard and actual quantity

  – The difference between the standard and actual unit cost

Variance Terminology

- Different variances are the responsibility of different managers
- Must separate total variances so that each manager can take appropriate action
- Quantity variances often called usage or efficiency variances
- Cost per unit of input variances often called price, rate, or spending variances

McGraw-Hill/Irwin — ©The McGraw-Hill Companies, Inc., 2002

Direct Labor Variances

- **Direct labor efficiency variance** is the quantity variance for direct labor
- The direct labor efficiency variance is the difference between standard hours allowed and actual hours worked
- **Direct labor rate variance** is the cost per unit of input variance
- The direct labor rate variance is the difference between actual and standard hourly pay rates

McGraw-Hill/Irwin — ©The McGraw-Hill Companies, Inc., 2002

Learning Objective 6

- What are the specific names assigned to variances for different product inputs?

McGraw-Hill/Irwin — ©The McGraw-Hill Companies, Inc., 2002

Variance Names

Input	Quantity	Cost per unit of Input
Raw materials	Usage	Price
Direct labor	Efficiency	Rate
Variable overhead	Efficiency	Spending

McGraw-Hill/Irwin   ©The McGraw-Hill Companies, Inc., 2002

General Variance Model

- Quantity variance =

$$\left[\begin{array}{c} \text{Standard} \\ \text{quantity} \\ \text{allowed} \end{array} - \begin{array}{c} \text{Actual} \\ \text{quantity} \\ \text{used} \end{array}\right] \times \begin{array}{c} \text{Standard} \\ \text{cost per} \\ \text{unit} \end{array}$$

- Cost per unit of input variance =

$$\left[\begin{array}{c} \text{Standard} \\ \text{quantity} - \\ \text{allowed} \end{array} \begin{array}{c} \text{Actual} \\ \text{quantity} \\ \text{used} \end{array}\right] \times \begin{array}{c} \text{Standard} \\ \text{cost per} \\ \text{unit} \end{array}$$

McGraw-Hill/Irwin   ©The McGraw-Hill Companies, Inc., 2002

Graphical Representation

Actual quantity used	Actual quantity used	Standard quantity allowed
X	X	X
Actual cost per unit	Standard cost per unit	Standard cost per unit

Cost per unit of Input variance	Quantity variance

McGraw-Hill/Irwin   ©The McGraw-Hill Companies, Inc., 2002

Variance Analysis Objectives

- Objective is to highlight deviations from planned results

- Want to eliminate unfavorable variances and capture favorable variances

- Need to analyze variances for each standard

- Usually raw materials usage variances and direct labor efficiency variances are reported frequently

McGrawHillIrwin ©The McGraw-Hill Companies, Inc., 2002

Raw Materials Purchase Variance

- Many firms calculate and report raw materials price variances at the time the materials are purchased rather than when they are used

- Modified purchase price variance:

Standard cost per unit	-	Actual cost per unit	X	Actual quantity purchased

McGrawHillIrwin ©The McGraw-Hill Companies, Inc., 2002

Learning Objective 7

- How do the control and analysis of fixed overhead variances and variable cost variances differ?

McGrawHillIrwin ©The McGraw-Hill Companies, Inc., 2002

Analysis of Fixed Overhead

- Analyzed differently from variable cost variances

- The focus is on the difference budgeted fixed overhead and actual fixed overhead expenditures

- This difference is divided into a budget variance and a volume variance

McGrawHillIrwin   ©The McGraw-Hill Companies, Inc., 2002

Fixed Overhead Volume Variance

- **Volume variance** is the difference between the amount of fixed overhead applied to production and that planned to be applied

- It is not appropriate to make per unit fixed overhead variance calculations because fixed costs do not behave on a per unit basis

McGrawHillIrwin   ©The McGraw-Hill Companies, Inc., 2002

Fixed Overhead Budget Variance

- The **budget variance** is the difference between budgeted fixed overhead for the period and the actual fixed overhead for the period

- Fixed overhead is difficult to control on a short-term basis

- But is a significant cost, so it receives management's attention

McGrawHillIrwin   ©The McGraw-Hill Companies, Inc., 2002

Learning Objective 8

- What are the alternative methods of accounting for variances?

McGraw-Hill/Irwin   ©The McGraw-Hill Companies, Inc., 2002

Accounting for Variances

- If the total of all of the variance is not significant, it is included with cost of goods sold in the income statement

- Standard costs also are released to cost of goods sold

- Therefore, cost of goods sold reports the actual cost of the items

- If variances are large, the variances are allocated between inventory and cost of goods sold

McGraw-Hill/Irwin   ©The McGraw-Hill Companies, Inc., 2002

CHAPTER 16

COST ANALYSIS FOR DECISION MAKING

McGraw-Hill/Irwin   ©The McGraw-Hill Companies, Inc., 2002

Learning Objectives

1. What are the meaning and application of the following "cost" terms: differential, allocated, sunk, and opportunity?
2. How are costs determined to be relevant for short-run decisions?
3. What is the special pricing decision when a firm is at full vs. idle capacity?

McGraw-Hill/Irwin   ©The McGraw-Hill Companies, Inc., 2002

Learning Objectives

4. What are the attributes of capital budgeting that make it a significantly different activity from operational budgeting?
5. Why is present value analysis appropriate in capital budgeting?
6. What is the concept of the cost of capital, and why is it used in capital budgeting?

McGraw-Hill/Irwin   ©The McGraw-Hill Companies, Inc., 2002

Learning Objectives

7. What are the uses of and differences between various capital budgeting techniques: net present value, present value ratio, and internal rate of return?

8. How are issues concerning estimates, income taxes, and the timing of cash flows and investments treated in the capital budgeting process?

9. How is the payback period of a capital expenditure project calculated?

Learning Objectives

10. How is the accounting rate of return of a project calculated, and how can it be used most appropriately?

11. Why are not all management decisions make strictly on the basis of quantitative analysis techniques?

Learning Objective 1

• What are the meaning and application of the following "cost" terms: differential, allocated, sunk, and opportunity?

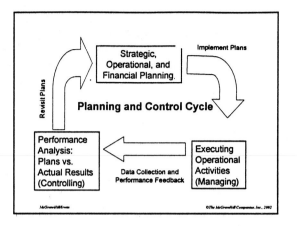

Cost Classifications for Other Analytical Purposes

- A **differential cost** is one that will differ according to the alternative activity selected

- **Allocated costs** are those that have been assigned to a product or activity using some sort of arithmetic process

  - Do not arbitrarily allocate costs because costs may not behave the way assumed in the allocation method

McGraw-Hill/Irwin   ©The McGraw-Hill Companies, Inc., 2002

Learning Objective 2

- How are costs determined to be relevant for short-run decisions?

McGraw-Hill/Irwin   ©The McGraw-Hill Companies, Inc., 2002

Relevant Costs

- Short-run decisions may affect only a few days or weeks

- Can involve:
  - The utilization of resources not otherwise active

  - The opportunity to reduce costs by adjusting the mix of resources

  - The ability to improve profits by further processing a product

McGraw-Hill/Irwin ©The McGraw-Hill Companies, Inc., 2002

Decision Analysis Classifications

- **Relevant costs** are:
  - Differential costs
  - Opportunity costs

- **Irrelevant costs** are:
  - Allocated costs
  - Sunk costs

McGraw-Hill/Irwin ©The McGraw-Hill Companies, Inc., 2002

Learning Objective 3

- What is the special pricing decision when a firm is at full vs. idle capacity?

McGraw-Hill/Irwin ©The McGraw-Hill Companies, Inc., 2002

Special Pricing Decision

- Firm is presented with a special offer for their product below the normal selling price

- Need to know where the firm is operating relative to capacity

- Need to consider only relevant costs – not allocated fixed costs

- Also must consider other factor such as affect on other customers

---

Learning Objective 4

- What are the attributes of capital budgeting that make it a significantly different activity from operational budgeting?

Capital Budgeting

- **Capital budgeting** is the process of analyzing proposed capital expenditures

- **Capital expenditures** are investments in plant, equipment, new products, etc.

- Want to determine if a large enough return on the investment can be generated over time

Capital Budgeting vs. Operational Budgeting

- The time frame being considered is different – longer – in capital budgeting

- Capital budgeting provides an overall blueprint to help the firm meet its long-term growth objectives

- Operational budget reflects firm's strategic plans to achieve current period profitability

Learning Objective 5

- Why is present value analysis appropriate in capital budgeting?

Investment Decision Special Considerations

- Investment decisions involve committing financial resources now in anticipation of a return in the future

- The time value of money must be considered due to the length of time involved

- Most firms have more investment opportunities than resources available

- Capital budgeting procedures help management identify favorable alternatives

Qualitative Factors

- Factors other than quantitative factors also must be considered

- Must consider things such as competitive risk, managements' personal goals, effects of selling additional stock if necessary

- Usually large expenditures require the approval of the board of directors

McGraw-Hill/Irwin ©The McGraw-Hill Companies, Inc., 2002

Learning Objective 6

- What is the concept of the cost of capital, and why is it used in capital budgeting?

McGraw-Hill/Irwin ©The McGraw-Hill Companies, Inc., 2002

Cost of Capital

- The **cost of capital** is the rate of return on assets that must be earned to permit the firm to meet its interest obligations and provide the expected return to owners

- Determining a firm's cost of capital is a complex process

- Cost of capital is a composite of borrowing costs and stockholder dividends and earnings' growth potential

McGraw-Hill/Irwin ©The McGraw-Hill Companies, Inc., 2002

Discount Rate

- The **cost of capital** is the discount rate used to determine the present value of the investment proposal being analyzed

- The **discount rate** is the interest rate at which future period cash flows are discounted

- Ranges from 10 – 20%

Capital Budgeting Techniques

- Methods that use present value analysis:
  - **Net present value (NPV) method**
  - **Internal rate of return (IRR) method**

- Methods that do not use present value analysis:
  - **Payback method**
  - **Accounting rate of return method**

Variables Used in Capital Budgeting Methods

- All methods use the amount to be invested

- The amount of cash generated by the investment is used in the NPV, IRR, and payback methods

- The accounting rate of return uses accrual accounting net income resulting from the investment

Learning Objective 7

- What are the uses of and differences between various capital budgeting techniques: net present value, present value ratio, and internal rate of return?

McGraw-Hill/Irwin   ©The McGraw-Hill Companies, Inc., 2002

Net Present Value

- Net present value method involves calculating the present value of the expected cash flows from the project using the cost of capital as the discount rate

- Then the net present value result is compared to the amount of investment required

- NPV often referred to as the hurdle rate

McGraw-Hill/Irwin   ©The McGraw-Hill Companies, Inc., 2002

Internal Rate of Return

- The IRR method solves for the actual rate of return that will be earned by the investment

- The IRR is the discount rate at which the present value of the cash flows from the project will equal the investment in the project

McGraw-Hill/Irwin   ©The McGraw-Hill Companies, Inc., 2002

Learning Objective 8

- How are issues concerning estimates, income taxes, and the timing of cash flows and investments treated in the capital budgeting process?

Some Analytical Considerations

- **Estimates** – the validity of the present value calculations will depend on the accuracy of the cash flow projections

- **Cash flows far in the future** – due to uncertainty, usually do not consider cash flows more than ten years in the future

- **Timing of cash flows within the year** – present value factors assume cash flows are received at the end of the year, but usually received throughout the year

---

Some More Analytical Considerations

- **Investment made over a period of time** – payments on the project may be made over a period of time, so interest on cash disbursements needs to be considered

- **Income tax effects of cash flows from the project** – must include income tax expenditures in cash flow projections

---

Still More Analytical Considerations

- **Working capital investment** – working capital needs will increase due to increases in accounts receivables and inventories and is treated like an additional investment

- **Least cost projects** – some expenditures are required by law, so need to choose the project with the lowest net cost

McGraw-Hill/Irwin   ©The McGraw-Hill Companies, Inc., 2002

_____

_____

_____

_____

_____

_____

_____

Learning Objective 9

- How is the payback period of a capital expenditure project calculated?

McGraw-Hill/Irwin   ©The McGraw-Hill Companies, Inc., 2002

_____

_____

_____

_____

_____

_____

_____

Payback Method

- The **payback method** is used to evaluate proposed capital expenditures by determining the length of time necessary to recover the amount of the investment

- Add up the cash inflows until the total equals the investment

- Then determine how many years it has taken to recover the investment

- Very simple method, but does not consider the time value of money

McGraw-Hill/Irwin   ©The McGraw-Hill Companies, Inc., 2002

_____

_____

_____

_____

_____

_____

_____

Learning Objective 10

- How is the accounting rate of return of a project calculated, and how can it be used most appropriately?

Accounting Rate of Return

- **Accounting rate of return** focuses on the impact of the investment project on the financial statements

- Done on a year-by-year basis

- Drawback is time value of money is not considered

- Often computed so stockholders will know the effect of the project on the financial statements

Learning Objective 11

- Why are not all management decisions make strictly on the basis of quantitative analysis techniques?

The Investment Decision

- Both quantitative and qualitative factors are considered
- Qualitative factors may include:
  - Commitment to a segment
  - Regulations that require an investment
  - Technological developments
  - Limited resources
  - Management's judgments about the accuracy of the estimates used

McGraw-Hill/Irwin   ©The McGraw-Hill Companies, Inc., 2002

Integration of Capital Budget with Operating Budgets

- Several aspects of the capital budget interact with the development of the operating budget:
  - Contribution margin increases and cost savings need to be included in the income statement budgets
  - Cash disbursements need to be included in the cash budget
  - Capital expenditures need to be included in the balance sheet budget

McGraw-Hill/Irwin   ©The McGraw-Hill Companies, Inc., 2002

EPILOGUE

ACCOUNTING –
THE FUTURE

McGrawHillIrwin   ©The McGrawHill Companies, Inc., 2002

Themes

1. Having a vision for the future
2. Competing in a global economy
3. Having insight and integrity
4. Committing to life-long learning
5. Becoming business Using technology effectively
6. partners
7. Turning vision into reality

McGrawHillIrwin   ©The McGrawHill Companies, Inc., 2002

Theme 1

- Using technology effectively

McGrawHillIrwin   ©The McGrawHill Companies, Inc., 2002

Accounting and Technology

- Computerized accounting systems "do" accounting today

- Accounting has evolved into a complex information system

- Inputs to the system will become increasingly automated

- Paperwork will become increasingly obsolete

McGraw-Hill/Irwin ©The McGraw-Hill Companies, Inc., 2002

Systems and Data Collection

- Technology can capture and record business events

- Accountants role is in the process of planning, analysis, design, implementation, use, and control of computerized transaction processing

- These transactions are captured in a database

McGraw-Hill/Irwin ©The McGraw-Hill Companies, Inc., 2002

Databases

- A **database management system** is a software application that stores data in a manner that allows users to interact with the data

- **Data warehouses** are large, refined collections of the organization's data resources

- **Data mining** technology allows organizations to search their database warehouses to find new knowledge about the organization

McGraw-Hill/Irwin ©The McGraw-Hill Companies, Inc., 2002

Retrieval of Information

- In the future there will be increased emphasis on tools that allow managers to retrieve data

- **Structured Query Language** is a language used to interact with databases

- Database tools can be used to provide information for external reporting

- Internet-based reporting will be done using **XBRL**

Theme 2

- Having a vision for the future

The Accounting Profession

- In 1998, the AICPA published the Vision Project which identified five core competencies that are essential for CPAs to survive in the next decade:
  - Communication and leadership skills
  - Strategic and critical thinking skills
  - Focus on the customer, client, and market
  - Interpretation of converging information
  - Being technologically adept

Theme 3

- Competing in a global economy

A Global Economy

- Today's business environment is global with a worldwide communication infrastructure

- Accounting standards vary widely from country to country

- The International Accounting Standards Committee is trying to harmonize accounting principles around the world

---

Theme 4

- Having insight and integrity

Insight and Integrity

- Enhanced skill sets will be needed by CPAs in the future

- A new professional designation is being proposed with four characteristics:
  - Global in reach
  - Based on wide range of disciplines
  - Bound by a global standard of ethics
  - Based on a global standard of competency with commitment to continuing learning

---

Theme 5

- Committing to life-long learning

Students of Accounting Information

- Business and accounting professionals must have a broad understanding of information technology and the role it plays in the new economy

- Students must understand what technology can and cannot do

Theme 6

- Becoming business partners

Becoming Business Partners

- Accounting professional must go beyond the traditional role of financial historians

- Transaction work and financial statement preparation now is done by computers

- The role is changing, but the perception will take longer to change

- Accounting work will be more analytical, more decision-oriented, less number crunching

Theme 7

- Turning vision into reality

Vision into Reality

- The future described is here – but not fully operational or widespread in application

- The technologies of the future will define accounting information needs in a global information age

McGraw-Hill/Irwin   ©The McGraw-Hill Companies, Inc., 2002